Part 2 MRCOG: 500 EMQs and SBAs

T0177002

Part 2 MRCOG: 500 EMQs and SBAs

Andrew Sizer
Shrewsbury and Telford Hospital NHS Trust and Keele University School of Medicine

Bidyut Kumar
Wrexham Maelor Hospital, Betsi Cadwaladr University Health Board

Guy Calcott
Shrewsbury and Telford Hospital NHS Trust

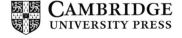
CAMBRIDGE
UNIVERSITY PRESS

CAMBRIDGE
UNIVERSITY PRESS

University Printing House, Cambridge CB2 8BS, United Kingdom

One Liberty Plaza, 20th Floor, New York, NY 10006, USA

477 Williamstown Road, Port Melbourne, VIC 3207, Australia

314–321, 3rd Floor, Plot 3, Splendor Forum, Jasola District Centre, New Delhi – 110025, India

79 Anson Road, #06-04/06, Singapore 079906

Cambridge University Press is part of the University of Cambridge.

It furthers the University's mission by disseminating knowledge in the pursuit of education, learning, and research at the highest international levels of excellence.

www.cambridge.org
Information on this title: www.cambridge.org/9781108709712
DOI: 10.1017/9781108627801

© Andrew Sizer, Bidyut Kumar and Guy Calcott 2019

This publication is in copyright. Subject to statutory exception and to the provisions of relevant collective licensing agreements, no reproduction of any part may take place without the written permission of Cambridge University Press.

First published 2019
Reprinted 2019

Printed in the United Kingdom by TJ International Ltd., Padstow Cornwall

A catalogue record for this publication is available from the British Library.

ISBN 978–1-108–70971-2 Paperback

Cambridge University Press has no responsibility for the persistence or accuracy of URLs for external or third-party internet websites referred to in this publication and does not guarantee that any content on such websites is, or will remain, accurate or appropriate.

Every effort has been made in preparing this book to provide accurate and up-to-date information that is in accord with accepted standards and practice at the time of publication. Although case histories are drawn from actual cases, every effort has been made to disguise the identities of the individuals involved. Nevertheless, the authors, editors and publishers can make no warranties that the information contained herein is totally free from error, not least because clinical standards are constantly changing through research and regulation. The authors, editors and publishers therefore disclaim all liability for direct or consequential damages resulting from the use of material contained in this book. Readers are strongly advised to pay careful attention to information provided by the manufacturer of any drugs or equipment that they plan to use.

Contents

Foreword

Membership of the Royal College of Obstetricians and Gynaecologists (MRCOG) is a highly regarded qualification throughout the world and confirms that the successful candidate has achieved a widely respected standard of knowledge, skills, attitudes and competencies in the practice of obstetrics and gynaecology. The award of MRCOG is made after successfully passing all three parts of the MRCOG examination. The Part 2 MRCOG is designed to test the skills necessary to pass from core clinical training (ST1–ST5) to higher specialist training (ST6 and ST7), and represents a significant hurdle in this transition.

This book of practice questions is an invaluable resource for candidates preparing for the Part 2 MRCOG examination. Written by experienced examiners and members of RCOG examination subcommittees, this book gives candidates the most relevant and authentic practice in preparation for the examination of all the currently available resources. The authors have vast expertise in writing examination questions and coaching candidates through courses, and therefore this book represents the most relevant examination preparation material available to date. The authors make very clear that this book should be used in addition to the standard revision resources as recommended by the RCOG but have helpfully referenced each and every explanation of the correct answer to enable the candidate to focus their revision of each particular topic.

This resource should become an essential part of examination preparation for all candidates attempting the Part 2 MRCOG examination.

Dr Lisa Joels MB ChB MD FRCOG FHEA
Chair of the RCOG Examination and Assessment Committee 2015–18

Preface

The current format of the Part 2 MRCOG examination is now well established with the change to written papers containing single best answer (SBAs) and extended matching questions (EMQs) commencing in March 2015.

The Part 2 MRCOG examination is primarily concerned with testing candidates' knowledge of the entire specialty of obstetrics and gynaecology as defined by the Royal College of Obstetricians and Gynaecologists (RCOG) curriculum.

The new Part 3 examination now provides the clinical assessment.

It is always preferable to enter an examination having had ample opportunity to practise the type of questions with which one will be faced. To this end, we have produced this book containing 250 SBA and 250 EMQ questions.

We have mapped the questions across all the modules of the curriculum that appear in the Part 2 MRCOG examination and have used the following sources as our primary references:

- RCOG guidelines
- National Institute for Health and Care Excellence (NICE) guidelines
- Articles in *The Obstetrician & Gynaecologist*.

The styles of the 500 questions are different, but this will mimic the actual examination, since numerous authors have contributed to the Part 2 MRCOG question bank.

In this book, we have tried to conform to the style of questions found in the Part 2 MRCOG examination but have deliberately separated the questions into the different modules of the syllabus. In this way, candidates will be able to test their knowledge in each of the modules after they have completed the necessary reading for that particular module. For each answer, we have provided a brief explanation and a reference to allow further or more in-depth reading of that subject. The explanations given here are not meant to replace the wider reading of the subject that is required to attain the level necessary to pass the Part 2 MRCOG examination.

Knowledge accumulates, practice alters and guidelines change. We will be grateful for feedback.

We hope that candidates for the Part 2 MRCOG will find this book helpful in their preparation for the Part 2 MRCOG examination.

Author profiles

Andrew Sizer

Andrew Sizer is a Consultant Obstetrician and Gynaecologist at the Shrewsbury and Telford Hospital NHS Trust and Senior Lecturer at Keele University School of Medicine. He is currently RCOG College Tutor for the Trust and Undergraduate Lead for Women's Health at the Shropshire campus for Keele University. Within the Postgraduate School of Obstetrics and Gynaecology in Health Education England, West Midlands, he is the Chair of Intermediate Training (ST3–5). He is the immediate past Chair of the Part 1 MRCOG examination committee and is current Chair of the standard setting committee and Honorary Deputy Director of Conferences at the RCOG. He was an examiner for the Part 2 MRCOG OSCE and is a current examiner for the Part 3 MRCOG clinical assessment. He is the lead author of two existing books for MRCOG examination preparation: *SBAs for the Part 1 MRCOG* (2012) and *Part 2 MRCOG: Single Best Answer Questions* (2016). He is also the developer of the andragOG.co.uk website, where a variety of other questions in a similar format are available.

Bidyut Kumar

Bid Kumar was appointed as a Consultant Obstetrician and Gynaecologist in 2001. He has been a RCOG tutor and a member of the Wales Deanery Specialty Training Committee. He is an honorary lecturer at Cardiff University Medical School and an honorary Senior Lecturer at Bangor University. He is a current Part 3 MRCOG examiner and has a number of current and former roles at the RCOG including the Part 2 course faculty, Part 2 MRCOG EMQ subcommittee and Green-top Guideline committee. He is Editor-in-Chief of *Ultrasound*, the journal of the British Medical Ultrasound Society, and an Associate Editor of the *The Obstetrician & Gynaecologist*. He actively contributes to the education and continued professional development of many healthcare professionals. Bid is an editor-author of *Fetal Medicine*, a textbook of the RCOG's Advanced Skills series (2016) and a co-author of *Tasks for Part 3 MRCOG Clinical Assessment* (2018). Bid also works for the National Guideline Alliance (NICE) as a topic lead for the review of many obstetric guidelines.

Guy Calcott

Guy Calcott is a newly appointed Consultant Obstetrician and Gynaecologist at the Shrewsbury and Telford Hospital NHS Trust with a special interest in high-risk obstetrics, maternal medicine and early pregnancy care. He qualified with a distinction in Medicine and Surgery from Imperial College School of Medicine in 2009 and a First Class Honours Bachelor of Science in Surgery and Anaesthesia. He completed foundation training and early obstetrics and gynaecology training at North West Thames before relocating to the West Midlands in 2013. He completed the MRCOG in 2015 and has been presenting and teaching on Part 2 MRCOG courses two to three times per year since 2016.

Acknowledgements

The authors would like to acknowledge the contribution of Mr Sujeewa Fernando, Consultant Obstetrician and Gynaecologist, Wrexham Maelor Hospital, to the questions included in module 18.

We would also like to thank the following doctors for being our 'proofreaders' during the first drafts of the manuscript and for their useful feedback: Dr Joanne Ritchie MRCOG, Dr Banchhita Sahu MRCOG, Dr Michael Algeo MRCOG, Dr James Castleman MRCOG, Dr Hector Georghiu MRCOG and Dr Pedro Melo MRCOG.

Normal ranges (non-pregnant) used in the MRCOG

Haematology

Haemoglobin (female):	115–160 g/l
Haematocrit (female):	37–47%
Total white cell count:	4.0×10^9–11.0×10^9/l
Platelets:	150×10^9–400×10^9/l

Clinical chemistry

Sodium:	135–145 mmol/l
Potassium:	3.5–5.2 mmol/l
Urea:	2.5–7.0 mmol/l
Creatinine:	60–120 μmol/l

Liver function

Albumin:	35–50 g/l
Total bilirubin:	0–22 μmol/l
Alkaline phosphatase:	40–130 IU/l
Alanine aminotransferase (ALT):	0–40 IU/l
γ-Glutamyl transferase:	0–75 U/l
Bile acids:	0–14 μmol/l

Endocrine

Thyroid-stimulating hormone (TSH):	0.35–5.5 mU/l
Free T4:	11–24 pmol/l
Follicle-stimulating hormone (FSH):	1–11 IU/l
Luteinising hormone (LH):	2–13 IU/l
Testosterone (female):	0.5–3.0 nmol/l
Testosterone (male):	8–30 nmol/l
Prolactin:	0–520 mU/l
Free androgen index:	0.5–6.5%
Sex hormone-binding globulin:	18–144 nmol/l

Cancer antigen 125 (CA125):	0–35 IU/ml

Please note: normal ranges can vary among laboratories.

Abbreviations

ACE	angiotensin-converting enzyme	FIGO	International Federation of Gynecology and Obstetrics
AED	anti-epileptic drug	FSH	follicle-stimulating hormone
AFP	α-fetoprotein	FSRH	Faculty of Sexual and Reproductive Healthcare
ALT	alanine transaminase		
AMH	anti-Müllerian hormone	GBS	group B *Streptococcus*
ARB	angiotensin-receptor blocker	GnRH	gonadotropin-releasing hormone
AREDV	absent or reversed end-diastolic velocity	GTG	Green-top Guideline
		HAART	highly active antiretroviral treatment
BASHH	British Association for Sexual Health and HIV	HBV	hepatitis B virus
BAUS	British Association of Urological Surgeons	hCG	human chorionic gonadotropin
BHIVA	British HIV Association	HELLP	haemolysis, elevated liver enzymes and low platelets
BMI	body mass index		
bpm	beats per minute	HFEA	Human Fertilisation and Embryology Authority
CBT	cognitive behavioural therapy	HIV	human immunodeficiency virus
cCTG	computerised CTG		
CEA	carcinoembryonc antigen	HRT	hormone replacement therapy
CI	confidence interval		
COCP	combined oral contraceptive pill	HSDD	hypoactive sexual desire disorder
CRP	C-reactive protein	HSG	hysterosalpingogram
CT	computerised tomography	HyCoSy	hystero-contrast-salpingography
CTG	cardiotocograph		
CTPA	computed tomography pulmonary angiography	IAP	intrapartum antibiotic prophylaxis
CXR	chest X-ray	ICSI	intracytoplasmic sperm injection
DCDA	dichorionic diamniotic		
DKA	diabetic ketoacidosis	IGFBP-1	insulin-like growth factor-binding protein-1
DVT	deep vein thrombosis		
EFW	estimated fetal weight	IUCD	intrauterine contraceptive device
EMQ	extended matching question		
ESHRE	European Society of Human Reproduction and Embryology	IVF	in vitro fertilisation
		LAM	lactational amenorrhoea method
FBC	full blood count	LAVH	laparoscopic-assisted vaginal hysterectomy
FBS	fetal blood sampling		
FGM	female genital mutilation	LDH	lactate dehydrogenase

LFT	liver function test	PCOS	polycystic ovarian syndrome
LH	luteinising hormone	PE	pulmonary embolism
LMWH	low-molecular-weight heparin	PET	positron emission tomography
LNG-IUS	levonorgestrel-releasing intrauterine system	PGE2	prostaglandin E2
		PID	pelvic inflammatory disease
MBRRACE	Mothers and Babies: Reducing Risk through Audits and Confidential Enquiries	PPROM	preterm prelabour rupture of membranes
		PTS	post-thrombotic syndrome
		PTSD	post-traumatic stress disorder
MCA	middle cerebral artery		
MCDA	monochorionic diamniotic	PUQE	pregnancy-unique quantification of emesis
MOGCT	malignant ovarian germ cell tumour	RCOG	Royal College of Obstetricians and Gynaecologists
MPA	medroxyprogesterone acetate		
MRKH	Mayer–Rokitansky–Kuster–Hauser	RMI	risk of malignancy index
		RCVS	reversible cerebral vasoconstriction syndrome
MRI	magnetic resonance imaging		
MRSA	methicillin-resistant *Staphylococcus aureus*	SBA	single best answer
		SGA	small for gestational age
NAAT	nucleic acid amplification test	ST	speciality trainee
		STV	short-term variation
NCEPOD	National Confidential Enquiry into Patient Outcome and Death	TCRE	transcervical resection of the endometrium
		TENS	transcutaneous electrical nerve stimulation
NHSLA	National Health Service Litigation Authority	TTP	thrombotic thrombocytopenic purpura
NICE	National Institute for Health and Care Excellence	TTTS	twin-to-twin transfusion syndrome
NSAID	non-steroidal anti-inflammatory drug	U&E	urea and electrolytes
		UDCA	ursodeoxycholic acid
NVP	nausea and vomiting in pregnancy	UKMEC	*UK Medical Eligibility Criteria for Contraceptive Use*
OASIS	obstetric anal sphincter injuries		
OHSS	ovarian hyperstimulation syndrome	UTI	urinary tract infection
		V/Q	ventilation/perfusion
OR	odds ratio	VBAC	vaginal birth after a caesarean
PAEC	progesterone receptor modulator-associated endometrial changes	VIN	vulval intraepithelial neoplasia
PAMG-1	placental α-microglobulin-1	VTE	venous thromboembolism
PCA	patient-controlled analgesia	WPBA	workplace-based assessment
PCO_2	partial pressure of carbon dioxide	WHO	World Health Organization

Introduction

Membership of the Royal College of Obstetricians and Gynaecologists (MRCOG) is an essential component of specialist training in obstetrics and gynaecology in the UK.

Possession of the MRCOG is also highly regarded by doctors working in other countries across the world, and many see the MRCOG as the 'gold standard' qualification in obstetrics and gynaecology.

Worldwide, there are over 16,000 Fellows and Members of the RCOG.

Format of the Part 2 MRCOG written examination

The Part 2 examination consists of two written papers with a short break (approximately 30–60 minutes) between them.

The two papers are identical in format and carry the same number of marks.

Each paper consists of 50 SBAs and 50 EMQs, but the weighting of the two question types is different, with the SBA component being worth 40% of the marks and the EMQ component 60%.

Each paper is of 3 hours' duration, but in view of the weighting, the RCOG recommends that candidates spend approximately 70 minutes on the SBA component and 110 minutes on the EMQ component. The only time warnings are 30 minutes and 10 minutes before the end of the examination, so candidates must take responsibility for their own time management. Candidates must also remember to allow enough time to transfer their answers onto the computer marking sheets, as there is no extra time to do this.

Traditionally, one paper is mainly obstetrics and the other mainly gynaecology, but there is no guarantee that this is this case, and, theoretically, any type of question or subject could appear in either paper.

Using this book

We hope that our 500 questions give a broad coverage of the syllabus and that you will find the different styles of question writing useful. However, as obstetrics and gynaecology is such a vast subject, it is not possible for 500 questions to cover every facet of the specialty.

Core modules 4 and 19 are not covered by the Part 2 examination so no questions on these two modules have been included.

Different modules cover different proportions of the curriculum. The two biggest modules in terms of subject area are antenatal care and gynaecological problems. These modules therefore have the greatest number of questions in the book, with other modules appropriately weighted according to their size.

We hope you find this book helpful as part of your examination preparation.

SBAs

1. A 28-year-old woman is admitted to the gynaecology ward with persistent nausea and vomiting in early pregnancy. Her serum urea and electrolytes are as follows:

Sodium	130 mmol/l
Potassium	3.0 mmol/l
Urea	4.3 mmol/l
Creatinine	100 µmol/l

What would be the most appropriate agent for electrolyte replacement therapy?
A. Intravenous potassium chloride 0.3% with glucose 5% solution
B. Intravenous potassium chloride 0.1% with sodium chloride 0.45% solution
C. Intravenous potassium chloride 0.3% with sodium chloride 0.9% solution
D. Oral potassium bicarbonate 500 mg with potassium acid tartrate 300 mg
E. Oral potassium chloride 600 mg tablets

2. What are the constituents of a litre of Hartmann's solution (in mmol)?

	Sodium	Potassium	Calcium	Bicarbonate	Chloride
A	131	5	2	29	111
B	136	7.7	2	30	120
C	140	7.5	5	29	111
D	145	5	2	29	150
E	150	7.5	10	29	111

3. A 34-year-old woman is admitted for an elective caesarean section. The woman is a known carrier of methicillin-resistant *Staphylococcus aureus* (MRSA).

    Which are the most appropriate prophylactic antibiotics to use in this situation?

	Cefuroxime	Clindamycin	Metronidazole	Teicoplanin	Vancomycin
A	✓	✓			
B		✓	✓		
C			✓	✓	
D				✓	✓
E	✓				✓

4. A 32-year-old multiparous woman has undergone an elective caesarean section under spinal anaesthesia at term. The spinal anaesthetic included intrathecal morphine.

    What is the minimum regime of postoperative clinical observations required for this woman?

    A. Continue observations every 30 minutes for 2 hours
    B. Continue observations every 30 minutes for 6 hours
    C. Continue observations every hour for 12 hours
    D. Continue observations every hour for 24 hours
    E. Continue observations every hour for 36 hours

5. Each year, there are approximately 700,000 deliveries in England and Wales.

    What proportion of these women will have undergone female genital mutilation (FGM)?

    A. 0.1%
    B. 1.5%
    C. 3%
    D. 4.5%
    E. 6%

EMQs
Options for questions 6–8

A	500–750 in 1000
B	250 in 1000
C	10 in 1000
D	7.5 in 1000
E	5 in 1000
F	2–3 in 1000
G	2 in 1000
H	1 in 1000
I	0.5 in 1000
J	0.2 in 1000

Each of the following clinical scenarios relates to the process of consenting for a treatment procedure. For each patient, select the single most appropriate option from the list above. Each option may be used once, more than once or not at all.

6. A 29-year-old woman attends the gynaecology clinic wishing to discuss laparoscopic sterilisation as she wants a permanent method of contraception. During counselling, she enquires about the risk of a serious complication.

7. A junior specialty trainee is about to see a 30-year-old woman who wishes to be sterilised. Only Filshie clips are used for sterilisation in the unit where he works. What is the failure rate that should be quoted?

8. A couple attend the clinic to discuss permanent methods of contraception. The woman is aged 35 years, has a body mass index (BMI) of 37 kg/m² and has had two caesarean sections. Her husband is aged 38 years. The woman is concerned about her risk of laparoscopic complications and wants her husband to consider a vasectomy. He enquires about the chance of late contraceptive failure after clearance for sterility is given following the vasectomy.

Options for questions 9 and 10

A	Amoxicillin 500 mg orally every 8 hours
B	Benzylpenicillin 3 g initially followed by 1.5 g 4 hourly
C	Cefalexin 500 mg orally every 8 hours
D	Ceftriaxone 2 g intravenous once daily
E	Clindamycin 900 mg intravenous every 8 hours
F	Co-amoxiclav 625 mg orally every 8 hours
G	Does not need antibiotic treatment
H	Gentamicin 4 mg/kg intravenous in three divided doses
I	Metronidazole 500 mg intravenous every 8 hours
J	Tetracycline 250 mg orally four times a day
K	Trimethoprim 200 mg orally twice daily
L	Vancomycin 1 g intravenous every 12 hours
M	Vancomycin 250 mg orally four times a day

Each of the following clinical scenarios relates to the choice of management for the prophylaxis or treatment of infection. For each patient, select the single most appropriate management from the list above. Each option may be used once, more than once or not at all.

9. A 24-year-old multiparous woman is in labour at 38 weeks' gestation. A high vaginal swab taken at 23 weeks of gestation grew group B *Streptococcus* in culture. She is severely allergic to penicillin.

10. A 67-year-old woman has been under treatment with various antibiotics for prolonged periods due to recurrent pneumonia. She now presents with diarrhoea and her stool culture has grown *Clostridium difficile*.

Answers
SBAs

1. Answer   **C**   Intravenous potassium chloride 0.3% with sodium chloride 0.9% solution

    Explanation
    Oral preparations are unsuitable in the given circumstances. Option B has a very low concentration of potassium unsuitable for treatment of hypokalaemia. Option A contains glucose, and glucose infusions should not be used because they can cause a further decrease in the plasma potassium concentration.

    Reference
    British National Formulary, 72. September 2016–March 2017.

2. Answer   **A**   Sodium 131 mmol, potassium 5 mmol, calcium 2 mmol, bicarbonate 29 mmol, chloride 111 mmol

    Explanation
    Hartmann's solution is one of the commonest intravenous infusions used in day-to-day practice on the ward. All grades of doctors must know its composition.

    Reference
    British National Formulary, 72. September 2016–March 2017.

3. Answer   **D**   Teicoplanin and vancomycin

    Explanation
    For MRSA carriers, teicoplanin or vancomycin should be used.

    Reference
    British National Formulary, 72. Bacterial infection. September 2016–March 2017.

4. Answer   **D**   Continue observations every hour for 24 hours

    Explanation
    For women who have had intrathecal opioids, there should be a minimum hourly observation of respiratory rate, sedation and pain scores for at least 12 hours for diamorphine and 24 hours for morphine.

    Reference
    NICE. Caesarean section. *NICE Clinial Guideline (CG 132)*. November 2011.

5. Answer   **B**   1.5%

    Explanation
    Since 2008, it has been estimated that 1.5% of women each year giving birth in England and Wales have undergone FGM.

    Reference
    Hussain S, Rymer J. Tackling female genital mutilation in the UK. *The Obstetrician & Gynaecologist* 2017;19:273–8.

EMQs

6. Answer **G** 2 in 1000

   Explanation
   Serious risks of laparoscopy include the overall risk of serious complications from diagnostic laparoscopy, which occur in approximately two women in every 1000.

7. Answer **F** 2–3 in 1000

   Explanation
   The longest period of available follow-up data for the most commonly used method in the UK, the Filshie clip, suggests a failure rate of 2–3 in 1000 procedures at 10 years.

8. Answer **I** 0.5 in 1000

   Explanation
   Individuals should be informed that a vasectomy has an associated failure rate and that pregnancy can occur several years after vasectomy. The contraceptive failure rate should be quoted as approximately 1 in 2000 (0.05%) after clearance has been given.

   ## References

   FSRH. Male and female sterilisation, *FSRH Clinical Guidance*. September 2014.
   RCOG. Diagnostic laparoscopy. *RCOG Consent Advice No. 2*. June 2017.

9. Answer **L** Vancomycin 1 g intravenous every 12 hours

   Explanation
   Provided a woman has not had a severe allergy to penicillin, a cephalosporin should be used. If there is any evidence of a severe allergy to penicillin, vancomycin should be used.

   ## Reference

   RCOG. Prevention of early-onset neonatal group B streptococcal disease. *RCOG GTG No. 36*. September 2017.

10. Answer **M** Vancomycin 250 mg orally four times a day

    Explanation
    For *C. difficile* infection, oral administration of vancomycin is more effective.

    ## Reference

    British National Formulary, 72. Infection. September 2016–March 2017.

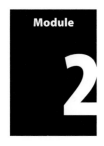

Module 2

Teaching and assessment

SBAs

11. In medical teaching, what is the single best determinant of expertise in a subject?

    A. Communication skills
    B. Knowledge
    C. Organisational skills
    D. Positive role modelling
    E. Technical ability

12. The SBAR format is commonly used on the delivery suite as a method to convey critical clinical information between different healthcare professionals.

    An ST5 telephones the consultant on call with the following communication.

    'Good evening, Dr Smith. This is John, the ST5, calling from the delivery suite. I have just been to see Mrs Jones who is in labour. The CTG is pathological. This woman is being monitored because of a previous stillbirth. I propose to take her to theatre for an immediate caesarean section.'

    What component of SBAR is missing from this communication?

    A. Achievement
    B. Action
    C. Alignment
    D. Alternatives
    E. Assessment

13. Which two tiers of Miller's pyramid are best assessed using workplace-based assessment tools?

	Knows	Knows how	Shows how	Does
A	✓	✓		
B	✓		✓	
C	✓			✓
D		✓	✓	
E			✓	✓

14. Which learning method is associated with the lowest retention of knowledge/information imparted?

   A. Lecture
   B. Practical demonstration
   C. Problem-based learning
   D. Reading a textbook
   E. Small group discussion

15. What is the only type of workplace-based assessment that has a summative role in obstetrics and gynaecology training?

   A. Case-based discussion
   B. Mini-Clinical Examination (Mini-CEX)
   C. Objective Structured Assessment of Technical Skills (OSATS)
   D. Reflective writing
   E. Team observation form

EMQs

Options for questions 16–18

A	Acceptability
B	Appraisability
C	Appraisal
D	Assessment
E	Construct validity
F	Content validity
G	Educational impact
H	Evaluation
I	Face validity
J	Feasibility
K	Feedback
L	Formative assessment
M	Reliability
N	Sensitivity
O	Specificity
P	Summative assessment
Q	Validity

The option list above relates to concepts, measurements and activities in medical education. For each of the following descriptions, what is the single most appropriate activity, measurement or concept that is being described? Each option may be used once, more than once or not at all.

16. The most important criterion for a quality assessment in medical education.

17. Pendleton's rules provide a model of delivering this kind of activity in medical education.

18. An activity that considers personal and educational development and is not measured against any set criteria.

Options for questions 19 and 20

A	Buzz groups
B	Case-illustrated learning
C	Circular questioning
D	Crossover groups
E	Fishbowls
F	Group round
G	Horseshoe groups
H	Problem-based learning
I	Snowball groups
J	Spiral groups

The option list above relates to methods of small group teaching. For each of the following descriptions, what is the single most appropriate small group teaching method that is being described? Each option may be used once, more than once or not at all.

19. The group is split into two, comprising an outer circle and an inner group. The outer circle members observe the inner group in the discussions in order to provide feedback.

20. The group is split into pairs and given a question or topic. Pairs combine to make a four, and then again to make an eight. The topics get more complex, and the groups of eight then feedback to the whole group.

Answers

SBAs

11. Answer **B** Knowledge

Explanation
Knowledge is the single best determinant of expertise in a subject. However, a practising obstetrician and gynaecologist also requires skills in communication, organisational ability, technical ability and teaching skills, as well as displaying the right attitude, to make them a good role model.

Reference
Duthie SJ, Garden AS. The teacher, the learner and the method. *The Obstetrician & Gynaecologist* 2010;12:273–80.

12. Answer **E** Assessment

Explanation
The SBAR format (situation, background, assessment, recommendation) is also of use in transmitting critical information and is now commonplace on many delivery suites:

> Situation: Good evening, Dr Smith. This is John, the ST5, calling from the delivery suite. I have just been to see Mrs Jones who is in labour. The CTG is pathological.
> Background: This woman is being monitored because of a previous stillbirth.
> Assessment: None.
> Recommendation: I propose to take her to theatre for an immediate caesarean section.

Reference
Jackson KS, Hayes K, Hinshaw K. The relevance of non-technical skills in obstetrics and gynaecology. *The Obstetrician & Gynaecologist* 2013;15:269–74.

13. Answer **E** 'Shows how' and 'Does'

Explanation
As the model for progression to mastery of a skill is sought, assessment is tailored to examine each of the pyramid's levels: Knows (knowledge), Knows how (competence), Shows how (performance) and Does (action). It has been suggested that WPBA assesses the top two levels of the pyramid: performance and action.

Reference
Parry-Smith W, Mahmud A, Landau A, Hayes K. Workplace-based assessment: a new approach to existing tools. *The Obstetrician & Gynaecologist* 2014;16:281–5.

14. Answer   **A**   Lecture

Explanation
Lectures result in only 5% retention.

Reference

Duthie SJ, Garden AS. The teacher, the learner and the method. *The Obstetrician & Gynaecologist* 2010;12:273–280

15. Answer   **C**   Objective Structured Assessment of Technical Skills (OSATS)

Explanation
All workplace-based assessments have a formative role. Only OSATS have a summative role.

Reference

Parry-Smith W, Mahmud A, Landau A, Hayes K. Workplace-based assessment: a new approach to existing tools. *The Obstetrician & Gynaecologist* 2014;16:281–5.

EMQs

16. Answer   **Q**   Validity

Explanation
Validity is the most important criterion of a quality assessment, i.e. the extent to which the assessment measures what it is intended to measure.

17. Answer   **K**   Feedback

Explanation
The two most widely accepted models of delivering feedback are Pendleton's rules and Silverman's agenda-led, outcome-based analysis. Both models provide a safe environment, thus reducing defensiveness and increasing constructiveness.

18. Answer   **C**   Appraisal

Explanation
Appraisal considers personal development as well as educational development and is not measured against any set criteria, nor does it contribute to a formal summative assessment. Appraisal is jointly developed by the trainee and trainer, and should be confidential and non-threatening.

Reference

Shehmar M, Khan KS. A guide to the ATSM in Medical Education. Article 2: assessment, feedback and evaluation. *The Obstetrician & Gynaecologist* 2010;12:119–25.

19. Answer   **E**   Fishbowls

    Explanation
    The usual fishbowl configuration has an inner group discussing an issue or topic while the outer group listens, looking for themes, patterns or soundness of argument, or uses a group behaviour checklist to give feedback to the group on its functioning. The roles may then be reversed.

20. Answer   **I**   Snowball groups

    Explanation
    Snowball groups (or pyramids) are an extension of buzz groups. Pairs join up to form fours, then fours to eights. These groups of eight report back to the whole group. This developing pattern of group interaction can ensure comprehensive participation, especially when it starts with individuals writing down their ideas before sharing them. To avoid students becoming bored with repeated discussion of the same points, it is a good idea to use increasingly sophisticated tasks as the groups gets larger.

Reference

Jaques D. Teaching small groups. *British Medical Journal* 2003;326:492–4.

IT, clinical governance and research

SBAs

21. A 45-year-old woman is admitted to the gynaecology ward for a planned hysterectomy for endometrial hyperplasia with atypia. A pregnancy test has not been carried out prior to theatre, and during the course of the laparotomy a mass is detected in the right fallopian tube that has an appearance suggestive of an unruptured ectopic pregnancy. A catheter specimen of urine is then used to perform a pregnancy test, which is found to be positive.

    What would be the correct course of action?

    A. Contact a colleague for a second opinion
    B. Contact the patient's partner for authorisation
    C. Continue with the hysterectomy including removal of the right tube
    D. Remove the right fallopian tube for histological confirmation
    E. Stop the surgery and reschedule

22. What type of consent is required for medical students performing pelvic examinations on anaesthetised women?

    A. Consent from the consultant responsible for the patient
    B. Formal consent is not required as this is part of clinical care
    C. Verbal consent from the woman
    D. Verbal consent witnessed by a member of the theatre staff
    E. Written consent

23. A pregnant woman attends the accident and emergency department with abdominal pain and vaginal bleeding. It is 7 weeks since her last menstrual period. She subsequently becomes tachycardic and hypotensive, and collapses. Plans are made to take her to the operating theatre.

    As per the National Confidential Enquiry into Patient Outcome and Death (NCEPOD), which category of intervention would this be?

    A. 1
    B. 2
    C. 3
    D. 4
    E. U

24. How many principal steps are there in an audit cycle?

    A. 3
    B. 4
    C. 5
    D. 6
    E. 7

25. Which phase of a clinical trial compares a new treatment with the current best available treatment?

    A. 0
    B. I
    C. II
    D. III
    E. IV

EMQs

Options for questions 26 and 27

A	Amniotic fluid embolism
B	Anaesthetic complications
C	Cardiac disease
D	Early pregnancy complications
E	Haemorrhage
F	Malignancy
G	Neurological disease
H	Pre-eclampsia
I	Sepsis
J	Suicide
K	Venous thromboembolism

From the list of options above, choose the single most appropriate cause of maternal death as published in the MBRRACE (Mothers and Babies: Reducing Risk through Audits and Confidential Enquiries) report of 2016. Each option may be chosen once, more than once or not at all.

26. The leading cause of indirect maternal death.

27. The leading cause of direct maternal death occurring within a year of the end of pregnancy.

Options for questions 28–30

A	Arrange meeting with Trust lawyer
B	Audit
C	High-risk case review
D	Refer case to Caldicott guardian
E	Refer concerns to Medical Director
F	Refer to coroner
G	Refer to multidisciplinary team meeting
H	Reflective entry in portfolio
I	Serious incident review
J	Service evaluation
K	Team debriefing session
L	Undertake root cause analysis

From the list of options above related to clinical governance, choose the single most appropriate initial course of action for each of the following scenarios. You may choose an option once, more than once or not at all.

28. A specialty trainee is collecting data for a research project. She has scanned copies of the patients' notes and saved these on an unencrypted memory stick. When she arrives home one evening, she cannot find the memory stick.

29. A fetal medicine specialist performs an amniocentesis at 17 weeks of gestation. Two days later, the woman has a miscarriage. The midwives feel that the particular specialist has a high miscarriage rate following antenatal invasive tests.

30. A woman is admitted for a planned caesarean section. During the course of the operation, she has a cardiac arrest and it is not possible to resuscitate her. She is thought to have had an amniotic fluid embolism.

Answers
SBAs

21. Answer   C   Continue with the hysterectomy including removal of the right tube

    Explanation
    A potentially viable pregnancy should not be terminated without the woman's consent and following the processes outlined in the 1967 Abortion Act. If a pregnancy is discovered at the start of a hysterectomy, including one for cancer, the operation should be rescheduled. An unexpected ectopic pregnancy should be removed. It is reasonable to presume that the woman would wish this and would wish the surgeon to act in favour of lifesaving treatment.

    Reference
    RCOG. Obtaining valid consent. *Clinical Governance Advice No. 6.* 2015.

22. Answer   E   Written consent

    Explanation
    Explicit consent of women is required for the presence of students:
    - During gynaecological and obstetric consultations
    - In operating theatres as observers and assistants
    - When performing a clinical pelvic examination.

    Written consent must be obtained for pelvic examination of anaesthetised women.

    Reference
    RCOG. Obtaining valid consent. *Clinical Governance Advice No. 6.* 2015.

23. Answer   A   Category 1

    Explanation
    NCEPOD categories are:

Category	Description	Time to theatre	Example
1	Immediate	Minutes	Haemorrhage
2	Urgent	Hours	Fracture
3	Expedited	Days	Tendon injury
4	Elective	Planned	Varicose veins

    Reference
    See the National Confidential Enquiry into Patient Outcome and Death (NCEPOD) website at www.ncepod.org.uk (accessed 25 July 2018).

24. Answer   C   5

Explanation
An audit can be considered to have five principal steps, commonly referred to as the audit cycle (see Figure 1 in the reference article):

1. Selection of a topic.
2. Identification of an appropriate standard.
3. Data collection to assess performance against the prespecified standard.
4. Implementation of changes to improve care if necessary.
5. Data collection for a second, or subsequent, time to determine whether care has improved.

Reference

RCOG. Understanding audit. *Clinical Governance Advice No. 5*. 2003.

25. Answer   D   III

Explanation
Traditionally, to introduce a drug into clinical practice, it passes through four phases:

- Phase I trials (20–80 people) to evaluate safety, determine a safe dosage range and identify side effects in a small group of people
- Phase II trials (100–300 people) to evaluate safety and to begin to determine efficacy
- Phase III trials (1000–3000 or more people if the chosen primary outcome measure has a low frequency, e.g. neonatal death) where it is compared to existing treatments
- Phase IV postmarketing studies to delineate additional information, such as the treatment risks, benefits and optimal use.

Reference

RCOG. Developing new pharmaceutical treatments for obstetric conditions. *Scientific Impact Paper No. 50*. 2015.

EMQs

26. Answer   C   Cardiac disease

Explanation
As in previous reports, cardiac disease remained the largest single cause of indirect maternal deaths in 2012–14.

27. Answer   J   Suicide

Explanation
The rate of maternal death by suicide remains unchanged since 2003, and maternal suicides are now the leading cause of direct maternal deaths occurring within a year after the end of pregnancy.

Reference

Knight M, Nair M, Tuffnell D, *et al.* (eds.) on behalf of MBRRACE-UK. *Saving Lives, Improving Mothers' Care: Surveillance of Maternal Deaths in the UK 2012–14 and Lessons Learned to Inform Maternity Care From the UK and Ireland Confidential Enquiries into Maternal Deaths and Morbidity 2009–14*. Oxford: National Perinatal Epidemiology Unit, University of Oxford, 2016.

28. Answer **D** Refer case to Caldicott guardian

Explanation
The Caldicott guardian is responsible for all breaches of personal data within a hospital Trust and should be informed immediately in such a case. Subsequent actions may include a serious incident review.

Reference

Roch-Berry C. What is a Caldicott guardian? *Postgraduate Medical Journal* 2003;79:516–18.

29. Answer **B** Audit

Explanation
Audit is a process whereby performance can be compared to a prespecified standard. All specialists will have some miscarriages after amniocentesis. An audit will determine if this doctor's performance is at odds with the expected rate.

The audit can be considered to have five principal steps, commonly referred to as the audit cycle (see answer to question 24 for details).

Reference

RCOG. Understanding audit. *Clinical Governance Advice No. 5*. 2003.

30. Answer **F** Refer to coroner

Explanation
A doctor may report the death to a coroner if:

- The cause of death is unknown
- The death was violent or unnatural
- The death was sudden and unexplained
- The person who died was not visited by a medical practitioner during their final illness
- The medical certificate is not available
- The person who died was not seen by the doctor who signed the medical certificate within 14 days before death or after they died
- The death occurred during an operation or before the person came out of anaesthetic
- The medical certificate suggests that the death may have been caused by an industrial disease or industrial poisoning.

Reference

See the gov.uk website at www.gov.uk/after-a-death/when-a-death-is-reported-to-a-coroner (accessed 25 July 2018).

Core surgical skills

SBAs

31. Which absorbable suture has the greatest tensile strength?

    A. Polydiaxonone (PDS)
    B. Polyglactic 910 (Vicryl rapide)
    C. Polyglactin (Vicryl)
    D. Polyglecaprone (Monocryl)
    E. Polyglycolic acid (Dexon)

32. What proportion of ureteric injuries are recognised intraoperatively during laparoscopic surgery?

    A. 10%
    B. 25%
    C. 33%
    D. 50%
    E. 67%

33. Which nerve is particularly susceptible to damage when self-retaining retractors are used in gynaecological surgery?

    A. Femoral nerve
    B. Genitofemoral nerve
    C. Iliohypogastric nerve
    D. Obturator nerve
    E. Pudendal nerve

34. During a primary caesarean section, at what point during the operation is a bladder injury most likely to occur?

    A. Closure of the uterine incision
    B. Delivery of the baby
    C. Dissection of bladder from the lower segment
    D. During catheterisation
    E. Entry into the peritoneal cavity

35. Taking all surgical procedures into consideration, which organism is most commonly implicated in inpatient surgical-site infections in England?

    A. *Enterobacteriaceae*
    B. *Enterococcus* spp.
    C. Methicillin-resistant *Staphylococcus aureus* (MRSA)
    D. *Pseudomonas* spp.
    E. *Staphylococcus aureus*

36. Urinary catheter size is identified by Charrière (Ch) or French gauge (Fg) or French (F).
    What does the gauge represent?

    A. External diameter
    B. Flow rate
    C. Internal diameter
    D. Length
    E. Volume of retaining balloon

37. What proportion of women in the UK have a body mass index (BMI) of >30 kg/m²?

    A. 6%
    B. 11%
    C. 16%
    D. 21%
    E. 26%

38. For an obese woman with no co-morbidities who has been unsuccessful in reducing her weight with dietary modification and exercise, what is the threshold BMI where bariatric surgery should be considered?

    A. 32 kg/m²
    B. 35 kg/m²
    C. 38 kg/m²
    D. 40 kg/m²
    E. 45 kg/m²

39. What is the overall approximate risk of serious complications from an abdominal hysterectomy?

    A. 1 in 100
    B. 2 in 100
    C. 3 in 100
    D. 4 in 100
    E. 5 in 100

40. A 45-year-old nulliparous woman who is otherwise fit and well attends for an outpatient hysteroscopy to investigate a potential polyp, which was suggested on an ultrasound scan.

    What pharmacotherapy would be recommended to reduce pain in the immediate postoperative period?

    A. Administration of a paracervical anaesthetic block
    B. Instillation of local anaesthetic gel into the cervical canal
    C. Oral non-steroidal anti-inflammatory drug (NSAID) an hour before the procedure
    D. Oral opiate analgesia 1 hour before the procedure
    E. Use of conscious sedation

41. What is the most appropriate suture material to repair the anorectal mucosa in a fourth-degree perineal tear?

    A. Polydiaxonone (PDS)
    B. Polyglactic 910 (Vicryl rapide)
    C. Polyglactin (Vicryl)
    D. Polyglecaprone (Monocryl)
    E. Polyglycolic acid (Dexon)

42. A 49-year-old woman is admitted to the gynaecology ward following an episode of significant vaginal bleeding due to a uterine fibroid. On examination, she is pale, well oriented and conscious.

    The observations are:

Temperature	37°C
Pulse	110 beats per minute
Blood pressure	90/60 mmHg
Urine	Small volume of very dark urine

    Which is the most appropriate intravenous fluid to be used for immediate resuscitation?

    A. Albumin 5%
    B. Dextrose 5%
    C. Sodium chloride 0.9%
    D. Sodium chloride 0.18%/4% glucose
    E. Sodium chloride 0.45%/4% glucose

43. A 25-year-old woman is admitted to the gynaecology ward following an evacuation of retained products of conception for a presumed molar pregnancy. On examination, her vital signs are within the normal range and stable. She is continuing to vomit and is unable to tolerate oral feed or fluids.

   What volume of fluid should be used for maintenance intravenous therapy?

   A. 5–9 ml/kg/day of fluid
   B. 10–14 ml/kg/day of fluid
   C. 15–19 ml/kg/day of fluid
   D. 20–24 ml/kg/day of fluid
   E. 25–29 ml/kg/day of fluid

44. What is the risk of major vessel injury with the Hasson (open) technique of laparoscopic entry?

   A. <0.1 in 1000
   B. 0.2 in 1000
   C. 0.5 in 1000
   D. 1 in 1000
   E. 2 in 1000

45. During primary entry with a force of 3 kg for gynaecological laparoscopy, what is the depth below the indented umbilicus with a peritoneal insufflation pressure of 25 mmHg?

   A. <4 cm
   B. 4–8 cm
   C. 9–13 cm
   D. 14–18 cm
   E. >18 cm

EMQs

Options for questions 46–50

A	Azygos artery of the vagina
B	Descending cervical artery, branch of the uterine artery
C	Descending cervical artery, branch of the internal iliac artery
D	Inferior epigastric artery, branch of the external iliac artery
E	Inferior epigastric artery, branch of the internal iliac artery
F	Inferior gluteal artery
G	Internal pudendal artery
H	Ovarian artery, branch of the abdominal aorta
I	Ovarian artery, branch of the internal iliac artery
J	Superior epigastric artery, branch of the internal thoracic artery
K	Superior gluteal artery
L	Superior vesical artery
M	Vaginal artery, branch of the descending cervical artery
N	Vaginal artery, branch of the internal iliac artery

Each of the following clinical scenarios relates to a pelvic surgical operative procedure. For each operative step, select the single most applicable option from the above list. Each option may be used once, more than once or not at all.

46. A 29-year-old woman has just undergone a knife cone biopsy of her cervix. Both angles of the cervix are bleeding profusely. A suture needs to be inserted to arrest this bleeding. Which blood vessel is the main contributor to this bleeding?

47. A 56-year-old woman is undergoing an abdominal hysterectomy for uterine fibroids. The surgeon attempts to open the vaginal vault to introduce a clamp on the vaginal angles and makes a stab wound in the midline on the vaginal vault just below and anterior to the cervix. The woman bleeds from the vaginal vault. Which vessel is the main source of this bleeding?

48. During a teaching session, the trainer is demonstrating the anatomy of pelvic blood vessels and demonstrates an artery that passes in between the piriformis and ischiococcygeus muscles and then round the sacrospinous ligament. There is another artery passing through the same space posteriorly. Which artery is this?

49. During a laparoscopic salpingectomy for ectopic pregnancy, the surgeon is about to introduce a lateral laparoscopic port on the left abdominal flank. The surgeon is trying to determine the correct position to make the incision and is looking for the course of a blood vessel. Which blood vessel is this?

50. A surgeon is demonstrating the anatomy of a pelvic blood vessel to a trainee. The surgeon traces the course of the internal iliac artery and identifies the largest branch. Which artery is this?

Answers
SBAs

31. Answer **A** Polydiaxonone (PDS)

Explanation
See Table 1 in the reference article.

Reference

Raghavan R, Arya P, Arya P, China S. Abdominal incisions and sutures in obstetrics and gynaecology. *The Obstetrician & Gynaecologist* 2014;16:13–18.

32. Answer **C** 33%

Explanation
There are seven types of ureteric injury, with transection the most commonly reported at laparoscopy. Only one-third of such injuries are recognised intraoperatively.

Reference

Minas V, Gul N, Aust T, Doyle M, Rowlands D. Urinary tract injuries in laparoscopic gynaecological surgery; prevention, recognition and management. *The Obstetrician & Gynaecologist* 2014;16:19–28.

33. Answer **A** Femoral nerve

Explanation
In a 10-year prospective study, Goldman *et al.* (1985; cited in the reference article) reported an 8% incidence of femoral neuropathy when self-retaining retractors were used during gynaecological surgery, compared with an incidence of <1% when not used.

Reference

Kuponiyi O, Alleemudder DI, Latunde-Dada A, Eedarapalli P. Nerve injuries associated with gynaecological surgery. *The Obstetrician & Gynaecologist* 2014;16:29–36.

34. Answer **E** Entry into the peritoneal cavity

Explanation
In a primary caesarean section, most bladder injuries occur during peritoneal entry, whereas in repeat caesarean sections, most occur during dissection of the bladder from the lower uterine segment (bladder flap creation).

Reference

Field A, Haloob R. Complications of caesarean section. *The Obstetrician & Gynaecologist* 2016;18:265–72.

35. Answer   **A**   *Enterobacteriaceae*

Explanation
The number of surgical-site infections with *Enterobacteriaceae* has continued to rise, whereas the proportion of other infections has remained static or fallen.

Reference
Public Health England. Surveillance of surgical site infections in NHS hospitals in England, 2016 to 2017. December 2017. Available from: www.gov.uk/phe (accessed 25 July 2018).

36. Answer   **A**   External diameter

Explanation
Catheter size is identified by Charrière (Ch) or French gauge (Fg) or French (F). These represent the external diameter of any catheter. It is recommended that the smallest size should be used, e.g. for women, use 12–14 Ch. However, a larger size should be used to drain and clear the urinary bladder when urine contains heavy grit (encrustation) or debris.

Reference
Aslam N, Moran PA. Catheter use in gynaecological practice. *The Obstetrician & Gynaecologist* 2014;16:161–8.

37. Answer   **E**   26%

Explanation
In the UK, 26% of women have a BMI of >30 kg/m^2.

Reference
RCOG. The role of bariatric surgery in improving reproductive health. *RCOG Scientific Impact Paper No. 17*. October 2015.

38. Answer   **D**   40 kg/m^2

Explanation
NICE guidelines recommend that bariatric surgery be considered when the BMI is 40 kg/m^2 or more, or for those with a BMI between 35 and 40 kg/m^2 in the presence of other co-morbidities and where other non-surgical methods have proven unsuccessful.

Reference
RCOG. The role of bariatric surgery in improving reproductive health. *RCOG Scientific Impact Paper No. 17*. October 2015.

39. Answer   **D**   4 in 100

Explanation
The overall risk of serious complications from an abdominal hysterectomy is approximately four women in every 100.

Reference
RCOG. Abdominal hysterectomy for benign conditions. *RCOG Consent Advice No. 4.* May 2009.

40. Answer   **C**   Oral non-steroidal anti-inflammatory drug (NSAID) an hour before the procedure

Explanation
Women without contraindications should be advised to consider taking standard doses of NSAIDs around 1 hour before their scheduled outpatient hysteroscopy appointment with the aim of reducing pain in the immediate postoperative period.
      Routine use of opiate analgesia before outpatient hysteroscopy should be avoided as it may cause adverse effects.
      Routine administration of intracervical or paracervical local anaesthetic is not indicated.

Reference
RCOG. Best practice in outpatient hysteroscopy. *RCOG GTG No. 59.* April 2011.

41. Answer   **C**   Polyglactin (Vicryl)

Explanation
Size 3-0 polyglactin (Vicryl) should be used to repair the anorectal mucosa as it may cause less irritation and discomfort than polydioxanone (PDS) sutures. When repair of the external and/or internal anal sphincter muscle is being performed, either monofilament sutures such as 3-0 PDS or modern braided sutures such as 2-0 polyglactin can be used with equivalent outcomes.

Reference
RCOG. The management of third- and fourth-degree perineal tears. *RCOG GTG No. 29.* June 2015.

42. Answer   **C**   Sodium chloride 0.9%

Explanation
If patients need intravenous fluid resuscitation, use crystalloids that contain sodium in the range 130–154 mmol/l, with a bolus of 500 ml over <15 minutes.

Reference
NICE. Intravenous fluid therapy in adults in hospital. *NICE Clinical Guidline (CG 174).* December 2013.

43. Answer **E** 25–29 ml/kg/day of fluid

Explanation
If patients need intravenous fluids for routine maintenance alone, restrict the initial prescription to: 25–30 ml/kg/day of water, approximately 1 mmol/kg/day of potassium, sodium and chloride and approximately 50–100 g/day of glucose to limit starvation ketosis.

Reference
NICE. Intravenous fluid therapy in adults in hospital. *NICE Clinical Guideline (CG 174)*. December 2013.

44. Answer **A** <0.1 in 1000

Explanation
Hasson reviewed a number of series using the open method and found no cases of major vessel injury and a rate of bowel injury of only 0.1%. In a meta-analysis of over 350,000 closed laparoscopic procedures, the risk of bowel damage was 0.4 in 1000 and of major vessel injuries was 0.2 in 1000.

Reference
RCOG. Preventing entry-related gynaecological laparoscopic injuries. *RCOG GTG No. 49*. May 2008.

45. Answer **B** 4–8 cm

Explanation
If a constant force of 3 kg is applied to the abdominal wall at the umbilicus to an abdominal cavity insufflated to a pressure of 10 mmHg, the depth under the 'indented' umbilicus is only 0.6 cm. When the same force is applied to an abdomen distended to 25 mmHg, the depth is 5.6 cm (range 4–8 cm).

Reference
RCOG. Preventing entry-related gynaecological laparoscopic injuries. *RCOG GTG No. 49*. May 2008.

EMQs

46. Answer **B** Descending cervical artery, branch of the uterine artery

47. Answer **A** Azygos artery of the vagina

48. Answer **F** Inferior gluteal artery

49. Answer **D** Inferior epigastric artery, branch of the external iliac artery

50. Answer **K** Superior gluteal artery

Reference
Standring S. (ed.) *Gray's Anatomy*, 40th edn. Churchill Livingstone, 2008.

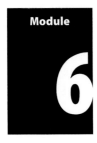

Module

6

Postoperative care

SBAs

51. A patient is referred to the gynaecology clinic for consideration of hysterectomy following a failed endometrial ablation.

    At what point should enhanced recovery planning start?

    A. Following discharge from hospital
    B. On admission
    C. Preoperative assessment clinic
    D. Upon completion of the operation
    E. With the initial referral

52. A woman has had a successful trial of forceps delivery under spinal anaesthetic.

    What is the minimum duration that the catheter should remain *in situ* to reduce the risk of asymptomatic bladder overfilling?

    A. 3 hours
    B. 6 hours
    C. 9 hours
    D. 12 hours
    E. 24 hours

53. A 48-year-old woman has undergone a midurethral tape procedure for stress urinary incontinence and is ready to be discharged.

    Within what time frame should she be seen as an outpatient to exclude tape erosion?

    A. 6 weeks
    B. 2 months
    C. 3 months
    D. 6 months
    E. 12 months

54. A patient is seen 2 weeks after a laparoscopic hysterectomy. An intraoperative bladder injury was noted and repaired laparoscopically by the urologist. A catheter has been left *in situ* for 2 weeks. A retrograde cystogram subsequently reports a leak from the bladder. The woman is clinically well.

    What is the most appropriate management?

    A. Leave catheter *in situ* and repeat cystogram in 1 week
    B. Perform cystoscopy to assess the defect
    C. Repeat laparoscopy and secondary repair
    D. Request a CT intravenous urogram to check ureters are not damaged
    E. Urgent urological review

55. A 38-year-old woman is admitted with nausea, vomiting and confusion following a transcervical resection of the endometrium (TCRE) for heavy menstrual bleeding. It is noted that the fluid deficit at the time of the procedure was 1.6 l.

    What is the single most important investigation?

    A. Chest X-ray
    B. CT of abdomen and pelvis
    C. Full blood count (FBC)
    D. Serum urea and electrolytes
    E. Ultrasound of the pelvis

56. A 49-year-old woman had a total abdominal hysterectomy and bilateral salpingo-oophorectomy for irregular menstrual bleeding and pelvic pain, related to previous diagnosis of endometriosis. Her immediate postoperative recovery was uneventful. Seven days later, she is readmitted with a vaginal loss of watery fluid and blood-stained urine.

    What is the most likely diagnosis?

    A. Detrusor overactivity
    B. Urinary retention with overflow
    C. Urinary tract infection
    D. Vaginal candidiasis
    E. Vesicovaginal fistula

57. Following surgery, how long should patients wait before they can shower?

    A. 24 hours
    B. 48 hours
    C. 72 hours
    D. 5 days
    E. 7 days

58. What is the most common type of postoperative infection following an emergency caesarean section?

    A. Endometritis
    B. Lower respiratory tract infection
    C. Upper respiratory tract infection
    D. Urinary tract infection
    E. Wound infection

59. Of women that develop pyrexia in the first 48 hours after gynaecological surgery, what proportion do not have an identifiable cause?

    A. 5%
    B. 10%
    C. 20%
    D. 40%
    E. 80%

60. Following a general anaesthetic, what is the most common cause of pyrexia in the immediate postoperative period?

    A. Lower respiratory tract infection
    B. Pulmonary atelectasis
    C. Upper respiratory tract infection
    D. Urinary tract infection
    E. Wound infection

EMQs

Options for questions 61–63

A	Common peroneal nerve
B	Femoral nerve
C	Genitofemoral nerve
D	Iliohypogastric nerve
E	Ilioinguinal nerve
F	Lateral cutaneous nerve of the thigh
G	Obturator nerve
H	Pudendal nerve
I	Radial nerve
J	Tibial nerve
K	Ulnar nerve

From the list of options above, which nerve is the most likely to be damaged in each of the following clinical scenarios? Each option may be used once, more than once or not at all.

61. Following a prolonged difficult hysterectomy for rectovaginal endometriosis, a 48-year-old woman makes a good postoperative recovery in hospital, although she did notice some altered sensation on the medial aspect of the thigh and calf. When she returns home a few days later, she is unable to climb the stairs.

62. Following a sacrospinous fixation procedure, a woman returns to hospital with worsening gluteal and vulval pain. The pain is worse when she sits down.

63. A woman with a body mass index (BMI) of 38 kg/m² is placed in the lithotomy position for a planned vaginal hysterectomy. It is necessary to hyperflex and abduct her thighs in order to gain adequate access. Postoperatively, she has foot drop and has altered sensation on the lateral aspect of her calf and the dorsum of her foot.

Options for questions 64–66

A	Bladder injury
B	Death
C	Femoral nerve damage
D	Haemorrhage requiring blood transfusion
E	Pelvic abscess
F	Prolapsed fallopian tube
G	Rectovaginal fistula
H	Surgical-site infection
I	Ureteric leakage
J	Ureteric ligation
K	Urinary tract infection
L	Vault haematoma
M	Vault prolapse
N	Venous thromboembolism
O	Vesicovaginal fistula
P	Wound dehiscence

The risk of an operation can be categorised into serious risk and frequently occurring risk. From the list of risks described above, choose the single most appropriate option for the scenario in question. Each option may be used once, more than once or not at all.

64. The most common serious risk of an abdominal hysterectomy.

65. The most common serious risk of vaginal surgery for prolapse.

66. The most common visceral injury (serious risk) associated with caesarean section.

Options for questions 67–70

A	Mixed respiratory and metabolic acidosis
B	Mixed respiratory and metabolic alkalosis
C	No derangement of acid–base balance
D	Primary metabolic acidosis
E	Primary metabolic acidosis with respiratory compensation
F	Primary metabolic alkalosis
G	Primary metabolic alkalosis with respiratory compensation
H	Primary respiratory acidosis
I	Primary respiratory acidosis with renal compensation
J	Primary respiratory alkalosis
K	Primary respiratory alkalosis with renal compensation

The list above describes some derangements of acid–base balance. For each of the following clinical scenarios, choose the single most appropriate derangement (if any) of acid–base balance. Each option may be used once, more than once or not at all.

67. Following a difficult hysterectomy for large fibroids, a woman remains in recovery for some time and needs several doses of morphine to maintain pain control. She returns to the ward with a patient-controlled analgesia device. When reviewed by a nurse 1 hour later, she has a low respiratory rate and low oxygen saturation on pulse oximetry.

    Her arterial blood gas results are:

pH	7.31
PCO$_2$	7.2 kPa
Base excess	+1.5

68. Following a difficult outpatient hysteroscopy, a woman becomes increasingly anxious. She is sweating and describes palpitations. Her ECG is normal.

    Her arterial blood gas results are:

pH	7.49
PCO$_2$	4.3 kPa
Base excess	−1.5

69. A woman with polycystic ovarian syndrome (PCOS) has been booked for laparoscopic ovarian drilling. Her periods are infrequent and she has been prescribed metformin to induce ovulation. Unbeknown to her gynaecologist, she has doubled the dose following internet advice that metformin induces weight loss. Following the laparoscopy, she is clammy and sweaty in the recovery area. She is tachypnoeic but her ECG is normal.

    Her results are:

Blood sugar	3.1 mmol/l
pH	7.28
PCO$_2$	3.9 kPa
Base excess	−2.8

70. A woman is admitted for surgical evacuation of the uterus following a presumed diagnosis of molar pregnancy. She has had severe vomiting for several days before the procedure. In the recovery area, she has ongoing vomiting, which is not controlled well by antiemetics. Eventually, a nasogastric tube is passed and attached to suction to keep her stomach empty. She continues to feel unwell with a low respiratory rate.

    Her arterial blood gas results are:

pH	7.49
PCO$_2$	6.2 kPa
Base excess	+2.5

Answers

SBAs

51. Answer **E** With the initial referral

Explanation
The GP has referred the patient with a request to consider an operation. The GP should therefore take steps to optimise the patient's health prior to them being seen in the clinic by checking for anaemia and treating accordingly, and optimising the treatment of any other underlying disease such as hypertension or diabetes.

Reference
RCOG. Enhanced recovery in gynaecology. *Scientific Impact Paper No. 36*. February 2013.

52. Answer **D** 12 hours

Explanation
There is considerable variation in practice in postpartum bladder management in the UK. Further research is needed to develop evidence-based guidelines. However, at a minimum, the first void should be measured, and if retention is a possibility, a postvoid residual should be measured to ensure that retention does not go unrecognised. Women who have had a spinal anaesthetic or an epidural that has been topped up for a trial should be offered an indwelling catheter for at least 12 hours postdelivery to prevent asymptomatic bladder overfilling, followed by fluid balance charts to ensure good voiding volumes.

Reference
RCOG. Operative vaginal delivery. *RCOG GTG No. 26*. February 2011.

53. Answer **D** 6 months

Explanation
Offer a follow-up appointment (including vaginal examination to exclude erosion) within 6 months to all women who have had continence surgery.

Reference
NICE. Urinary incontinence in women: management. *NICE Clinical Guideline (CG171)*. September 2013.

54. Answer **A** Leave catheter *in situ* and repeat cystogram in 1 week

Explanation
Ideally, bladder repairs should be watertight, and leakage from the suture line should be tested (e.g. with methylene blue or indigo carmine). A bladder catheter must be inserted and continuous postoperative bladder drainage should be allowed for 2 weeks. The above two measures (watertight closure and indwelling catheter) will improve healing and reduce the risk of subsequent vesicovaginal fistula formation. Prior to catheter removal, complete repair without leakage

should be confirmed by retrograde cystography. If contrast escape is noted, then the catheter should be left *in situ* and the test repeated in 1 week.

Reference

Minas V, Gul N, Aust T, Doyle M, Rowlands D. Urinary tract injuries in laparoscopic gynaecological surgery; prevention, recognition and management. *The Obstetrician & Gynaecologist*, 2014;16:19–28.

55. Answer   **D**   Serum urea and electrolytes

Explanation

Transurethral resection syndrome, a well-recognised complication with first-generation ablative techniques, occurs secondary to glycine overload. Glycine overload can cause hyponatraemia and hyperammonaemia, congestive heart failure, haemolysis, coma and, in rare instances, death. Fluid balance is a fundamental part of the operative set-up and requires careful measurement of input and output. A deficit level of 1.5 l should be used as a reference mark for when to stop the procedure, because deficits below this level are not associated with metabolic changes of transurethral resection syndrome (hyponatraemia and hyperammonaemia).

Nausea, vomiting, headache and confusion are early signs of hyponatraemia, and therefore urea and electrolytes should give the answer.

Reference

Saraswat L, Cooper K. Surgical management of heavy menstrual bleeding: part 1. *The Obstetrician & Gynaecologist* 2017;19:37–45.

56. Answer   **E**   Vesicovaginal fistula

Explanation

The presenting complaint of a constant watery loss per vaginam is suggestive of a fistula. Blood-stained urine would also indicate some kind of urinary tract injury.

57. Answer   **B**   48 hours

Explanation

Advise patients that they may shower safely 48 hours after surgery.

Reference

NICE. Surgical site infections: prevention and treatment. *NICE Clinical Guideline (CG74)*. Updated February 2017.

58. Answer   **A**   Endometritis

Explanation

Wound infection and endometritis are the commonest sites of postoperative infection, although the urinary tract, respiratory tract and nervous system must also be considered. The risk of sepsis is, unsurprisingly, higher for emergency compared with elective caesarean section. A 2014 Cochrane review suggested a rate of wound infection of 97 in 1000 and 68 in 1000 for emergency and elective caesarean section, respectively; for endometritis, the rates were 184 in 1000 versus 39 in 1000, respectively.

Reference

Field A, Haloob R. Complications of caesarean section. *The Obstetrician & Gynaecologist* 2016;18:265–72.

59. **Answer**   **D**   40%

Explanation
Almost 40% of women with fever in the first 48 hours postoperatively do not have an identifiable cause.

Reference

Read M, James M. Immediate postoperative problems following gynaecological surgery. *The Obstetrician & Gynaecologist* 2002;4:29–34.

60. **Answer**   **B**   Pulmonary atelectasis

Explanation
Postoperative pyrexia is commonly caused by pulmonary atelectasis developing during general anaesthetic. If the pyrexia persists beyond 36 hours, a chest X-ray may be required.

Reference

Read M, James M. Immediate postoperative problems following gynaecological surgery. *The Obstetrician & Gynaecologist* 2002;4:29–34

EMQs

61. **Answer**   **B**   Femoral nerve

Explanation
Gynaecological surgery is the most common contributor to iatrogenic femoral nerve injury, and abdominal hysterectomy is mostly responsible for this.
 Femoral neuropathy presents with weakness of hip flexion and adduction and knee extension.

62. **Answer**   **H**   Pudendal nerve

Explanation
The pudendal nerve (S2–S4) exits the pelvis initially through the greater sciatic foramen below the piriformis. Importantly, it runs behind the lateral third of the sacrospinous ligament and ischial spine alongside the internal pudendal artery and immediately re-enters the pelvis through the lesser sciatic foramen to the pudendal canal (Alcock's canal). This nerve is susceptible to entrapment injuries during sacrospinous ligament fixation as it runs behind the lateral aspect of the sacrospinous ligament. The patient will report postoperative gluteal, perineal and vulval pain, which worsens in the seated position if the nerve is damaged.

63. Answer **A** Common peroneal nerve

Explanation
Foot drop is reported when the common peroneal nerve is injured, along with paraesthesia over the calf and dorsum of the foot.

Reference
Kuponiyi O, Alleemudder DI, Latunde-Dada A, Eedarapalli P. Nerve injuries associated with gynaecological surgery. *The Obstetrician & Gynaecologist* 2014;16:29–36.

64. Answer **D** Haemorrhage requiring blood transfusion

Explanation
Haemorrhage requiring blood transfusion occurs in 23 women in every 1000 abdominal hysterectomies (common). All other serious risks are uncommon or rare.

Reference
RCOG. Abdominal hysterectomy for benign conditions. *RCOG Consent Advice No. 4*. May 2009.

65. Answer **D** Haemorrhage requiring blood transfusion

Explanation
The risk of excessive bleeding requiring transfusion or a return to theatre is 2 in every 100 (common).

Reference
RCOG. Vaginal surgery for prolapse. *RCOG Consent Advice No. 5*. October 2009.

66. Answer **A** Bladder injury

Explanation
The risk of bladder injury is 1 in every 1000 (rare). The risk of ureteric injury is 3 in every 10,000 (rare).

Reference
RCOG. Caesarean section. *RCOG Consent Advice No. 7*. October 2009.

67. Answer **H** Primary respiratory acidosis

Explanation
This is a primary respiratory acidosis demonstrated by low pH and elevated partial pressure of carbon dioxide (PCO_2). Base excess is normal. Opiates cause respiratory depression and in an acute situation there is inadequate time for renal compensation.

68. Answer   **J**   Primary respiratory alkalosis

Explanation
A highly anxious woman is likely to hyperventilate. This can quickly result in primary respiratory alkalosis and this is reflected in the blood gases. As this is an acute event, there is no time for renal compensation.

69. Answer   **E**   Primary metabolic acidosis with respiratory compensation

Explanation
This woman is potentially taking high doses of metformin, which is associated with lactic acidosis. She will have been starved for her operation, which has led to hypoglycaemia. Her acidotic state has resulted in increased ventilation in an attempt to correct her acid–base disturbance via respiratory compensation (hence the reason the PCO_2 is low).

70. Answer   **G**   Primary metabolic alkalosis with respiratory compensation

Explanation
This woman has metabolic alkalosis with respiratory compensation. Prolonged vomiting causes depletion of sodium and potassium. The kidney retains sodium at the expense of hydrogen ions, so the pH falls. Respiratory compensation occurs when ventilation is slowed, so the PCO_2 rises.

Reference

Barrett K, Brooks H, Boitano S, Barman S. *Ganong's Review of Medical Physiology*, 25th edn. Lange Medical Books, 2015.

Surgical procedures

SBAs

71. A woman presents with pelvic pain and swelling and is found to have a 10 cm ovarian cyst. Imaging suggests that this is a dermoid cyst. A laparoscopy is performed, but the surgeon decides the cyst is too large to remove laparoscopically and converts the procedure to a mini-laparotomy.

    When compared with a laparoscopic procedure, which two factors will be reduced?

	Operative time	Postoperative discomfort	Rate of spillage of cyst contents	Recovery time
A	✓	✓		
B		✓	✓	
C			✓	✓
D	✓		✓	
E		✓		✓

72. During the course of an outpatient hysteroscopy with a 3 mm hysteroscope, a doctor finds that he has perforated the uterus. Patient observations are stable and there is no evidence of any bleeding.

    What is the most appropriate management?

    A. Admit for 24-hour observation and intravenous antibiotics
    B. Arrange an urgent laparoscopy
    C. Arrange an urgent laparotomy
    D. Insert a urinary catheter and observe for 12 hours
    E. Reassure and discharge

73. When comparing open myomectomy and hysterectomy for the surgical management of a fibroid uterus, which perioperative complication is more likely with hysterectomy?

    A. Haemorrhage
    B. Infection
    C. Ovarian artery thrombosis
    D. Return to theatre
    E. Visceral damage (bladder or bowel)

74. Which laparoscopic procedure appears to be associated with the highest rate of bladder injury?
   A. Laparoscopic-assisted vaginal hysterectomy (LAVH)
   B. Laparoscopic myomectomy
   C. Laparoscopic ovarian cystectomy
   D. Subtotal laparoscopic hysterectomy
   E. Total laparoscopic hysterectomy

75. A 30-year-old woman with a normal body mass index (BMI) has a laparoscopic ovarian cystectomy for a persistent 6 cm simple ovarian cyst. Preoperative tumour markers were normal. The tissue is placed in a retrieval bag.
   Ideally, through which port/incision should the tissue be removed?
   A. Lateral laparoscopic port
   B. McBurney's point incision
   C. Midline suprapubic port
   D. Palmer's point incision
   E. Umbilical port

76. A 26-year-old woman has had a laparoscopic salpingotomy for an ectopic pregnancy. She enquires about the future risk of another ectopic pregnancy.
   What is the risk of having a subsequent ectopic pregnancy following a salpingotomy?
   A. 2%
   B. 8%
   C. 14%
   D. 20%
   E. 26%

77. Which operative procedure for vaginal vault prolapse results in the lowest rate of recurrence?
   A. High uterosacral ligament suspension
   B. High ventrofixation
   C. Modified McCall culdoplasty
   D. Open abdominal sacrocolpopexy
   E. Sacrospinous fixation

78. A 32-year-old multiparous woman with a previous history of caesarean section is now at 38 weeks of gestation with placenta praevia. She has been admitted for caesarean section. At the time of signing the consent form, she enquires about the chances of an emergency hysterectomy.
   What is the risk of emergency hysterectomy for this woman?
   A. 27%
   B. 37%
   C. 47%
   D. 57%
   E. 67%

79. A woman has a laparoscopy for suspected appendicitis at 18 weeks of gestation. What is the maximum recommended intra-abdominal pressure during the procedure?
    A. 8 mmHg
    B. 10 mmHg
    C. 12 mmHg
    D. 15 mmHg
    E. 20 mmHg

80. What is the risk of bladder injury during caesarean section?
    A. 0.001%
    B. 0.005%
    C. 0.01%
    D. 0.05%
    E. 0.1%

EMQs

Options for questions 81–85

A	40 in 100 women
B	26 in 100 women
C	20 in 100 women
D	10 in 100 women
E	8 in 100 women
F	6 in 100 women
G	4 in 100 women
H	2 in 100 women
I	1 in 100 women
J	<1 in 100 women

Each of the following clinical scenarios relates to a woman who is about to have a surgical procedure. For each risk described, select the single most appropriate incidence from the list above. Each option may be used once, more than once or not at all.

81. A 35-year-old woman is about to have a diagnostic laparoscopy for chronic pelvic pain. She is concerned because her sister had an umbilical hernia following a similar operation done through the umbilicus. During the consenting process, she enquires about her risk of developing a hernia through the site of entry.

82. A 35-year-old woman has suffered a third-degree perineal tear following her first delivery at term. Following repair of the tear, the doctor wishes to prescribe antibiotics to her. She is apprehensive about taking antibiotics because of her previous history of *Clostridium difficile* infection related to antibiotic use during an episode of pneumonia. She asks about her risk of perineal infection following this repair.

83. A 36-year-old multiparous woman has just had a repair of her third-degree perineal tear following a forceps delivery. What is the incidence of faecal urgency following such repair?

84. A 63-year-old woman attends the gynaecology clinic for counselling and consenting for vaginal hysterectomy for prolapse. She has an 'unusual antibody' in her blood and is worried about the prospect of needing blood transfusion during surgery. She enquires about the risk of intraoperative blood transfusion.

85. A 27-year-old woman has suffered a missed miscarriage at 10 weeks of gestation. Following a period of expectant management she has started bleeding and now wants to have a surgical evacuation of the uterus. She enquires about the risk of retained products of conception following the surgical evacuation.

Options for questions 86–90

A	A small vertical incision starting at the base of the umbilicus
B	A transverse incision at the lower edge of the umbilicus
C	A vertical incision in the skin below the umbilicus
D	A small incision 3 cm below the left costal margin in the midclavicular line
E	Insertion into the abdomen at 90° to the skin with the operating table horizontal
F	Insertion into the abdomen at 90° to the skin with the operating table in Trendelenburg position
G	Insertion into abdomen at 45° to the skin aiming at the pelvis
H	Insertion into abdomen at 45° to the skin with the operating table horizontal
I	Insertion at 90° to the horizontal plane irrespective of the position of the operating table
J	Move Veress needle from side to side to ensure that the tip is free inside the abdomen
K	Reduce abdominal distension pressure to 15 mmHg
L	Rotate the laparoscope through 360° to visualise and exclude any adhesion of bowel
M	Start insufflation if intra-abdominal pressure remains between 10 and 15 mmHg
N	Tilt the operation table to the Trendelenburg position
O	Tilt operation table to the Trendelenburg position before starting to inflate the abdomen
P	Visualisation of inferior epigastric artery

Each of the following clinical scenarios relates to actions or manoeuvres during laparoscopic entry. For each patient, select the single most appropriate action from the option list above. Each option may be used once, more than once or not at all.

86. A 32-year-old woman with a previous history of midline laparotomy is about to undergo laparoscopy. A senior specialty trainee (ST5) is teaching a junior specialty trainee (ST2) to introduce a laparoscope into the abdomen. The junior trainee enquires about the exact location of incision in order to introduce the Veress needle.

87. A senior trainee doctor is about to introduce the Veress needle into the abdomen of a 19-year-old woman who is undergoing laparoscopy for chronic pelvic pain. The doctor has made an incision. Which is the most appropriate manoeuvre while the doctor introduces the Veress needle?

88. A senior trainee doctor is performing a diagnostic laparoscopy for a 42-year-old woman with a history of chronic pelvic pain. The doctor has successfully introduced the laparoscope through the primary port. Which is the next most appropriate manoeuvre?

89. A surgeon needs to introduce secondary ports for performing a laparoscopic excision of a simple ovarian cyst in a 36-year-old multiparous woman. The laparoscope is in the correct position through the primary port. A 360° view inside the abdomen is normal. What is the next most important step?

90. A junior specialty trainee (ST2) is doing her first laparoscopy on a nulliparous woman with a BMI of 29 kg/m² but no other known risk factors in her history. The ST2 doctor has checked all the equipment and must now make an incision for introduction of the Veress needle. Where is the most appropriate site on the woman's abdomen to place the incision?

Options for questions 91–95

A	Approximation of the uterosacral ligaments using continuous sutures, so as to obliterate the peritoneum of the posterior cul-de-sac as high as possible (McCall culdoplasty)
B	Attaching the uterosacral and cardinal ligaments to the vaginal cuff and high circumferential obliteration of the pouch of Douglas
C	Colposuspension along with sacrocolpopexy
D	Colpocleisis
E	Delayed absorbable polydioxanone sutures for uterosacral ligament suspension
F	Placing concentric purse string sutures around the cul-de-sac to include the posterior vaginal wall, the right pelvic side wall, the serosa of the sigmoid and the left pelvic side wall
G	Sacrospinous fixation
H	Subtotal hysterectomy
I	Transvaginal mesh procedure
J	Uterosacral ligament suspension with delayed absorbable sutures
K	Uterosacral ligament suspension with permanent sutures

Each of the following clinical scenarios relates to a surgical procedure. For each scenario, select the single most appropriate procedure from the list of options above. Each option may be used once, more than once or not at all.

91. An 89-year-old single woman with hypertension and chronic obstructive lung disease presents with a procidentia. She is taking warfarin for atrial fibrillation. Examination reveals a small atrophic uterus with the vaginal vault lying outside the introitus. What is the most appropriate surgical technique for her prolapse?

92. A 68-year-old woman is undergoing vaginal hysterectomy for a second-degree uterine prolapse. The woman has a cystocele but no enterocele. What technique should be adopted to reduce the chances of posthysterectomy vaginal vault prolapse?

93. A 65-year-old woman presents with a complete vaginal vault prolapse. She has been informed that, following an operation for correcting her prolapse, occult urinary incontinence may become manifest in the form of stress urinary incontinence. She asks whether any operative procedure could help reduce her chances of urinary incontinence after surgery. Which is the most appropriate technique?

94. A 70-year-old woman has just had a vaginal hysterectomy for procidentia. During closure, the vaginal vault descends to just beyond the introitus. What procedure should be considered to reduce her chances of posthysterectomy vaginal vault prolapse?

95. A 59-year-old woman is undergoing a hysterectomy for uterine fibroids. The surgeon wishes to reduce the woman's risk of having a posthysterectomy vaginal vault prolapse. Which is the most appropriate procedure?

Answers
SBAs

71. Answer **D** Operative time and rate of spillage of cyst contents

    Explanation
    Randomised trials have shown that, while mini-laparotomy is associated with
    a significant increase in minor postoperative discomfort and recovery time,
    and more pain and the need for analgesia, as well as more aesthetic concerns,
    operative times are shorter and rates of intraperitoneal spillage are significantly
    reduced.

    Reference
    Stavroulis A, Memtsa M, Yoong W. Methods for specimen removal from the peritoneal
    cavity after laparoscopic excision. *The Obstetrician & Gynaecologist* 2013;15:26–30.

72. Answer **A** Admit for 24 hours observation and intravenous antibiotics

    Explanation
    See Figure 1 in the reference article.

    Reference
    Shakir F, Diab Y. The perforated uterus. *The Obstetrician & Gynaecologist* 2013;15:256–61.

73. Answer **E** Visceral damage (bladder or bowel)

    Explanation
    Women who have a laparotomy for hysterectomy or myomectomy show similar
    surgical complications, such as haemorrhage, unintended repeat surgery and
    rehospitalisation, while bladder and bowel injuries are more frequent with a
    hysterectomy.

    Reference
    Younas K, Hadoura E, Majoko F, Bunkheila A. A review of evidence-based management of
    uterine fibroids. *The Obstetrician & Gynaecologist* 2016;18:33–42.

74. Answer **A** Laparoscopic-assisted vaginal hysterectomy (LAVH)

    Explanation
    Certain types of procedures, such as LAVH, appear to be associated with a higher
    frequency of bladder injury compared with others.

    Reference
    Minas V, Gul N, Aust T, Doyle M, Rowlands D. Urinary tract injuries in laparoscopic
    gynaecological surgery; prevention, recognition and management. *The Obstetrician &
    Gynaecologist* 2014;16:19–28.

75. Answer **E** Umbilical port

    Explanation
    Removing tissue in a tissue retrieval bag via the umbilical port has been
    investigated in a randomised and large prospective trial. Removal of benign

ovarian masses via the umbilical port should be utilised where possible, as this results in less postoperative pain and a quicker retrieval time. Avoidance of extending accessory ports is beneficial in reducing postoperative pain, as well as reducing the incidence of incisional hernia and the incidence of epigastric vessel injury. It also leads to improved cosmesis.

Reference

RCOG. Management of suspected ovarian masses in premenopausal women. *RCOG GTG No. 62.* December 2011.

76. Answer **B** 8%

Explanation
A multicentre randomised controlled trial on 446 women with a laparoscopically confirmed tubal ectopic pregnancy and a healthy contralateral tube found that the cumulative ongoing pregnancy rate was 60.7% after salpingotomy and 56.2% after salpingectomy. Persistent trophoblasts occurred more frequently in the salpingotomy group (14 (7%) versus 1 (<1%); relative risk 15.0, 95% confidence interval (CI) 2.0–113.4). A repeat ectopic pregnancy occurred in 18 women (8%) in the salpingotomy group and 12 (5%) in the salpingectomy group (relative risk 1.6, 95% CI 0.8–3.3). It was concluded that in women with a tubal ectopic pregnancy and a healthy contralateral tube, salpingotomy does not significantly improve fertility prospects compared with salpingectomy.

Reference

RCOG. Diagnosis and management of ectopic pregnancy. *RCOG GTG No. 21.* November 2016.

77. Answer **D** Open abdominal sacrocolpopexy

Explanation
Open abdominal sacrocolpopexy is associated with significantly lower rates of recurrent vault prolapse, dyspareunia and postoperative stress urinary incontinence when compared with sacrospinous fixation. However, this is not reflected in significantly lower reoperation rates or higher patient satisfaction. There is limited evidence on the effectiveness of robotic sacrocolpopexy; therefore, it should only be performed in the context of research or prospective audit following local governance procedures. High uterosacral ligament suspension should only be offered as first-line management in women with posthysterectomy vaginal vault prolapse within the context of research or prospective audit following local governance procedures.

Reference

RCOG. Post hysterectomy vaginal vault prolapse. *RCOG GTG No. 46.* July 2015.

78. Answer **A** 27%

Explanation
In women with placenta praevia and a previous caesarean section, the risk of emergency hysterectomy is up to 27 in 100 women (very common). In women

with an abnormally adherent placenta (e.g. placenta accreta), the woman should be advised that hysterectomy is highly likely.

Reference

RCOG. Caesarean section for placenta praevia. *RCOG Consent Advice No. 12.* December 2010.

79. Answer   **C**   12 mmHg

Explanation
Surgery on a pregnant patient with acute appendicitis should include a left lateral tilt to avoid aortocaval compression, avoidance of uterine or cervical manipulation or instrumentation, and limiting intra-abdominal pressure to <12 mmHg.

Reference

Weston P, Moroz P. Appendicitis in pregnancy: how to manage and whether to deliver. *The Obstetrician & Gynaecologist* 2015;17:105–10.

80. Answer   **E**   0.1%.

Explanation
Serious risks of caesarean section include: bladder injury (1 in 1000, rare), ureteric injury (3 in 10,000, rare) and death (approximately 1 in 12,000, very rare).

Reference

RCOG. Caesarean section. *RCOG Consent Advice No. 7.* October 2009.

EMQs

81. Answer   **J**   <1 in 100 women

82. Answer   **E**   8 in 100 women

83. Answer   **B**   26 in 100 women

84. Answer   **H**   2 in 100 women

85. Answer   **G**   4 in 100 women

References

RCOG. Vaginal surgery for prolapse. *RCOG Consent Advice No. 5.* October 2009.
Repair of third and fourth degree perineal tear following childbirth. *RCOG Consent Advice No. 9.* June 2010.
Diagnostic laparoscopy. *RCOG Consent Advice No. 2.* June 2017.
Surgical management of miscarriage and removal of persistent placental or fetal remains. *RCOG Consent Advice No. 10 (joint with AEPAU).* January 2018.

86. Answer **D** A small incision 3 cm below the left costal margin in the midclavicular line

Explanation
The rate of adhesion formation at the umbilicus may be up to 50% following midline laparotomy and 23% following low transverse incision. The umbilicus may not, therefore, be the most appropriate site for primary trocar insertion following previous abdominal surgery. The most usual alternative site is in the left upper quadrant, where adhesions rarely form, although even this may be inappropriate if there has been previous surgery in this area or splenomegaly. The preferred point of entry is 3 cm below the left costal margin in the midclavicular line (Palmer's point).

87. Answer **E** Insertion into abdomen at 90° to the skin with the operating table horizontal

Explanation
The Veress needle should be sharp, with a good and tested spring action. A disposable needle is recommended, as it will fulfil these criteria. The operating table should be horizontal (not in the Trendelenburg tilt) at the start of the procedure. The abdomen should be palpated to check for any masses and for the position of the aorta before insertion of the Veress needle.
     The lower abdominal wall should be stabilised in such a way that the Veress needle can be inserted at right angles to the skin and it should be pushed in just sufficiently to penetrate the fascia and the peritoneum.

88. Answer **L** Rotate the laparoscope through 360° to visualise and exclude any adhesion of bowel

Explanation
Once the laparoscope has been introduced through the primary cannula, it should be rotated through 360° to check visually for any adherent bowel. If this is present, it should be closely inspected for any evidence of haemorrhage, damage or retroperitoneal haematoma.

89. Answer **N** Tilt the operation table to the Trendelenburg position

Explanation
The Trendelenburg position helps the bowel to move out of the pelvis to allow safe entry of secondary ports. All such ports should be introduced under direct vision.

90. Answer **A** A small vertical incision starting at the base of the umbilicus

Explanation
In most circumstances, the primary incision for laparoscopy should be vertical from the base of the umbilicus (not in the skin below the umbilicus). Care should be taken not to incise so deeply as to enter the peritoneal cavity.

Reference

RCOG. Preventing entry-related gynaecological laparoscopic injuries. *RCOG GTG No 49.* May 2008.

91. Answer **D** Colpocleisis

Explanation

Colpocleisis is a useful procedure in women with serious co-morbidities. Colpocleisis is a safe and effective procedure that can be considered for frail women and/or women who do not wish to retain sexual function.

92. Answer **A** Approximation of the uterosacral ligaments using continuous sutures, so as to obliterate the peritoneum of the posterior cul-de-sac as high as possible (McCall culdoplasty)

Explanation

A small randomised controlled trial compared vaginal Moschcowitz-type operation, McCall culdoplasty and peritoneal closure of the cul-de-sac as preventative measures against the development of an enterocele. It showed that McCall culdoplasty was more effective than vaginal Moschcowitz or simple closure of the peritoneum in preventing an enterocele at the 3-year follow-up.

93. Answer **C** Colposuspension along with sacrocolpopexy

Explanation

Colposuspension performed at the time of sacrocolpopexy is an effective measure to reduce postoperative symptomatic stress urinary incontinence in previously continent women.

94. Answer **G** Sacrospinous fixation

Explanation

Sacrospinous fixation at the time of vaginal hysterectomy should be considered when the vault descends to the introitus during closure.

95. Answer **B** Attaching the uterosacral and cardinal ligaments to the vaginal cuff and high circumferential obliteration of the pouch of Douglas

Explanation

Suturing the cardinal and uterosacral ligaments to the vaginal cuff at the time of hysterectomy is effective in preventing posthysterectomy vaginal vault prolapse following both abdominal and vaginal hysterectomies.

Reference

RCOG. Post-hysterectomy vaginal vault prolapse. *RCOG GTG No. 46.* July 2015.

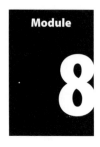

Module 8

Antenatal care

SBAs

96. A 32-year-old woman is seen for preconception counselling. She has a history of breast cancer and has just completed a course of tamoxifen.
    How long should she wait before she can try to conceive?

    A. 4 weeks
    B. 6 weeks
    C. 3 months
    D. 6 months
    E. 1 year

97. A 38-year-old woman is seen in antenatal clinic at 12 weeks of gestation. She has a body mass index (BMI) of 37 kg/m² and does not regularly undertake exercise.
    What would the recommendation be with regard to starting exercise in pregnancy in order to control her weight?

    A. Do not recommend initiating exercise in pregnancy
    B. Gentle exercise for 60 minutes per day
    C. Gentle exercise for 60 minutes three times per week
    D. Moderate aerobic exercise for 15 minutes per day three times per week
    E. Moderate aerobic exercise for 30 minutes per day

98. A 27-year-old woman attends for her pregnancy dating scan. She is unsure of the date of her last menstrual period. The following fetal measurements are obtained:

Crown–rump length	86 mm
Biparietal diameter	18 mm
Head circumference	100 mm
Femur length	12 mm
Abdominal circumference	67 mm

Which of these measurements should be used to date the pregnancy?

    A. Abdominal circumference
    B. Biparietal diameter
    C. Crown–rump length
    D. Femur length
    E. Head circumference

99. A 42-year-old woman is seen in the booking clinic in her first pregnancy. She has a history of chronic hypertension and is taking methyldopa. She is white Caucasian with a BMI of 24 kg/m².

     What daily dose of vitamin D should be recommended for her throughout this pregnancy?

     A. 400 units
     B. 800 units
     C. 1000 units
     D. 1200 units
     E. 1500 units

100. With regard to the routine anomaly scan in pregnancy, what threshold of nuchal-fold measurement should trigger a referral to a fetal medicine specialist?

     A. 6 mm
     B. 7 mm
     C. 8 mm
     D. 9 mm
     E. 10 mm

101. In an uncomplicated pregnancy, how often should auscultation of the fetal heart be performed by the midwifery team?

     A. Every 2 weeks from 24 weeks
     B. Every 3 weeks from 24 weeks
     C. Every 4 weeks from 24 weeks
     D. Every appointment after 20 weeks
     E. Only when requested by the mother

102. A 37-year-old pregnant woman is seen in the clinic at 42 weeks of gestation. She declines an offer of induction of labour, wanting to keep things 'as natural as possible'.

     What management should be offered?

     A. Daily cardiotocograph (CTG), twice weekly amniotic fluid volume assessment and umbilical artery Doppler
     B. Daily CTG and twice weekly umbilical artery Doppler
     C. Daily CTG, weekly amniotic fluid volume assessment and umbilical artery Doppler
     D. Twice weekly CTG and amniotic fluid volume assessment
     E. Twice weekly CTG, amniotic fluid volume assessment and umbilical artery Doppler

103. A 26-year-old woman is seen for her antenatal booking appointment. She was in a road traffic accident 10 years ago and has a spinal cord transection at the level of T11 and is paraplegic. What additional complication is she at risk of when compared with women with lower spinal cord injuries?

A. Autonomic dysreflexia
B. Inability to perceive labour pains
C. Late preterm labour
D. Malpresentation at term
E. Ventilatory dysfunction

104. A woman is seen at 24 weeks of gestation in the joint obstetric and mental health clinic with a psychiatrist. She has been referred by the community midwife because of the woman's concerns after watching her sister give birth. She recounts her sister having a very traumatic forceps delivery followed by a massive haemorrhage, describing 'blood everywhere'. She is diagnosed with severe anxiety and post-traumatic stress disorder (PTSD). She is requesting an elective caesarean section.

What intervention would be most appropriate?

A. Citalopram
B. Cognitive behavioural therapy (CBT)
C. Facilitated self-help
D. Fluoxetine
E. Offer an elective caesarean section at 39 weeks

105. A 32-year-old woman is seen in the antenatal clinic. She is 16 weeks pregnant and is planning to go to Tanzania for a safari in 4 weeks. She enquires about malaria prophylaxis.

What would be the primary recommendation?

A. Ensure she takes chemoprophylaxis and continues after the trip
B. Keep her skin covered as much as possible
C. Postpone the trip if possible
D. Take standby treatment (quinine) with her
E. Use insecticide-impregnated mosquito nets at night

106. A woman with a monochorionic diamniotic (MCDA) twin pregnancy at 25 weeks of gestation has been diagnosed with severe twin-to-twin transfusion syndrome (TTTS) and has been referred to the regional centre.

What is the recommended first-line management, assuming no contraindications to any treatment?

A. Laser ablation of placental vessels
B. Radiofrequency ablation of placental vessels
C. Selective amnioreduction
D. Selective feticide via cord coagulation
E. Septostomy

107. A woman presents to the obstetric triage unit with reduced fetal movements at 27 weeks of gestation. She has a monochorionic twin pregnancy. A CTG is performed. It is normal in the presenting twin but shows a bradycardia in twin 2. Both twins have a cephalic presentation. Preparations are made for emergency delivery, but during this time in the antenatal ward, the fetal heart of twin 2 stops. An ultrasound examination confirms the absence of a fetal heartbeat in twin 2.

    What is the most appropriate action?

    A. Administer steroids and commence induction of labour when appropriate
    B. Administer steroids and deliver by caesarean section when appropriate
    C. Continue with a category 1 caesarean section
    D. Postpone delivery and perform a detailed ultrasound scan after 4 weeks
    E. Postpone delivery and perform fetal MRI after 4 weeks

108. A woman is referred from the antenatal clinic with reduced fetal movements at 29 weeks of gestation. Computerised CTG (cCTG) is normal with a short-term variation (STV) of 8 ms. Ultrasound shows an estimated fetal weight plotting below the 10th centile, with reversed end-diastolic flow in the umbilical artery. Middle cerebral artery (MCA) Doppler and ductus venosus Doppler are normal. She was given a course of steroids 2 weeks previously for a threatened preterm labour.

    What is the recommended management?

    A. Category 2 caesarean section
    B. Daily CTG and deliver if STV is <5 ms
    C. Daily Dopplers and deliver if ductus venosus becomes abnormal
    D. Daily Dopplers and deliver if MCA Doppler becomes abnormal
    E. Immediate induction of labour

109. A 28-year-old woman in her first pregnancy is in the antenatal clinic at 12 weeks of gestation. She has a history of female genital mutilation (FGM). On examination, she has type 3 FGM, and the vaginal orifice admits one finger only.

    What would be the recommended management?

    A. Anterior episiotomy at the time of delivery
    B. Deinfibulation as soon as possible
    C. Deinfibulation at 20 weeks
    D. Deinfibulation at 28 weeks
    E. Deinfibulation in early labour

110. What is the most common adverse obstetric problem in a pregnancy complicated by unexplained antepartum haemorrhage?

    A. Fetal growth restriction
    B. Oligohydramnios
    C. Premature rupture of membranes
    D. Preterm delivery
    E. Stillbirth

111. Which obstetric complication has a significantly increased likelihood in women who have undergone bariatric surgery?

    A. Delivery by caesarean section
    B. Gestational diabetes
    C. Large-for-gestational-age fetus
    D. Pre-eclampsia
    E. Small-for-gestational-age (SGA) fetus

112. What is the incidence of vasa praevia in women who have had successful in vitro fertilisation (IVF) treatment?

    A. 1 in 10 pregnancies
    B. 1 in 30 pregnancies
    C. 1 in 100 pregnancies
    D. 1 in 300 pregnancies
    E. 1 in 1000 pregnancies

113. A woman at 36 weeks of gestation has prelabour rupture of membranes. She has a temperature of 40°C and is hypotensive with a systolic blood pressure of 85 mmHg. She has a diffuse macular rash and gives a history of vomiting and diarrhoea. Blood tests reveal a significantly raised creatinine level, and her bilirubin level is also raised.

    What single additional feature would confirm a diagnosis of staphylococcal toxic shock?

    A. Coagulopathy with platelets $<100 \times 10^9/l$
    B. Desquamation of the palms and soles
    C. Isolation of *Staphylococcus* from a throat swab
    D. Lactate >4 mmol/l
    E. Oropharyngeal hyperaemia

114. A woman is seen in antenatal clinic at 39 weeks. It is her first pregnancy and she is concerned about continuing the pregnancy beyond her estimated date of delivery. She is asking about a membrane sweep.

    When should a first membrane sweep be offered for this woman?

    A. A membrane sweep is not routinely offered
    B. Offer a membrane sweep at 39 weeks onwards
    C. Offer a membrane sweep at 40 weeks onwards
    D. Offer a membrane sweep at 41 weeks onwards
    E. Offer a membrane sweep prior to formal induction of labour

115. What is the earliest gestational age at which amniocentesis can be performed?

    A. 12 weeks
    B. 13 weeks
    C. 14 weeks
    D. 15 weeks
    E. 16 weeks

116. A 29-year-old woman at 33 weeks of gestation presents with a 24-hour history of symptoms suggestive of preterm prelabour rupture of membranes (PPROM).
    Which initial test should be performed to confirm a diagnosis of PPROM?

    A. Nitrazine test
    B. Speculum examination of the vagina
    C. Test vaginal fluid for insulin-like growth factor-binding protein-1 (IGFBP-1)
    D. Test vaginal fluid for placental α-microglobulin-1 (PAMG-1)
    E. Ultrasound scan for assessment of amniotic fluid volume

117. A 33-year-old woman has just had her second normal vaginal delivery. She is a known group B *Streptococcus* (GBS) carrier, and received the loading dose of benzylpenicillin 30 minutes prior to delivery. She is otherwise low risk obstetrically and the baby was born in good condition.
    What initial management of the neonate would be recommended?

    A. 48-Hour admission
    B. Increased observations for 12 hours
    C. Take bloods and treat if C-reactive protein (CRP) raised or cultures positive
    D. Treat as normal
    E. Treat with prophylactic antibiotics

118. A 40-year-old woman in her first pregnancy attends antenatal clinic for advice at 10 weeks of gestation. She is fit and healthy and has no significant past medical history. She asks whether it is safe to drink alcohol in pregnancy. Her preferred drink is red wine.
    What would be the recommended upper limit of amount of wine that she could drink in this pregnancy?

    A. 80 ml one to two times per week
    B. 100 ml one to two times per week
    C. 120 ml one to two times per week
    D. 140 ml one to two times per week
    E. 160 ml one to two times per week

119. A new screening test is being assessed in a university antenatal clinic looking at the ability of a raised serum level of substance X to detect Down's syndrome in women over 45 years of age. One hundred women are entered into the trial and 12 test positive for raised serum levels of substance X. Of these 12, eight are subsequently found to have babies with Down's syndrome. From the 100 women, there are ten cases of Down's syndrome in total.
    What is the sensitivity of elevated substance X to detect Down's syndrome in these women?

    A. 4%
    B. 8%
    C. 10%
    D. 12%
    E. 80%

120. Which three classes of antihypertensive drugs appear to be associated with an increased risk of congenital malformations?

	Angiotensin-converting enzyme (ACE) inhibitors	Angiotensin-receptor blockers (ARB)	β-Blockers	Calcium-channel blockers	Thiazides
A	✓	✓	✓		
B		✓	✓	✓	
C			✓	✓	✓
D	✓			✓	✓
E	✓	✓			✓

121. For any potentially sensitising event, rhesus D-negative, previously non-sensitised women should receive a minimum dose of 500 IU anti-D immunoglobulin (Ig) intramuscularly within 72 hours of the event, regardless of whether the woman has already received routine antenatal anti-D Ig prophylaxis at 28 weeks. Any additional dose of anti-D Ig needed is guided by a test of maternal blood for fetomaternal haemorrhage.

The dose calculation is based on which formula?

A. 100 IU anti-D Ig/ml of fetal red blood cells
B. 125 IU anti-D Ig/ml of fetal red blood cells
C. 150 IU anti-D Ig/ml of fetal red blood cells
D. 175 IU anti-D Ig/ml of fetal red blood cells
E. 200 IU anti-D Ig/ml of fetal red blood cells

122. A 28-year-old woman in her second pregnancy has a booking blood test at 14 weeks of gestation that shows the presence of anti-K antibody at a titre of 1 in 16. What is the most appropriate action?

A. Immediate maternal blood test for fetal genotyping for K antigen
B. Maternal blood test for fetal genotyping for K antigen after 20 weeks of gestation
C. Measure titre every 2 weeks until 28 weeks
D. Measure titre every 4 weeks until 32 weeks
E. Paternal blood test for genotyping for K antigen

123. What is the optimum method of screening for chromosomal abnormality in a monochorionic twin pregnancy at 13 weeks of gestation?

A. Amniocentesis
B. Combined screening test
C. Non-invasive prenatal testing
D. Nuchal translucency measurement
E. Quadruple test

124. At her booking visit with a midwife, a 27-year-old woman is offered haemoglobinopathy screening using the Family Origin Questionnaire. She is deemed to be at low risk.

    What value of mean corpuscular haemoglobin would trigger laboratory screening?

    A. <27 pg
    B. 27–29 pg
    C. 30–32 pg
    D. 33–35 pg
    E. >35 pg

125. What is the primary reason that serological screening for hepatitis B is routinely offered to all pregnant women?

    A. To help cross-match blood for transfusion as and when needed
    B. To implement antenatal intervention to decrease the risk of mother-to-child transmission
    C. To implement postnatal intervention to decrease the risk of mother-to-child transmission
    D. To reduce the risk of infecting healthcare providers
    E. To treat the mother to avoid worsening of hepatitis B disease

126. A high level of vitamin A intake in the first trimester of pregnancy may be harmful to the fetus and poses a risk of teratogenicity.

    What is the recommended upper limit of daily intake of vitamin A in early pregnancy?

    A. 500 µg
    B. 600 µg
    C. 700 µg
    D. 800 µg
    E. 900 µg

127. A 27-year-old multiparous woman had spontaneous rupture of membranes at 37 weeks of gestation. She is a carrier of group B *Streptococcus* (GBS) as detected on a vaginal swab in the second trimester.

    What is the most appropriate management?

    A. Await spontaneous labour and use intrapartum antibiotic prophylaxis (IAP)
    B. Offer one dose of prophylactic antibiotic before elective caesarean delivery
    C. Offer induction of labour after 24 hours and IAP
    D. Offer induction of labour at 41 weeks and IAP
    E. Offer induction of labour immediately and IAP

128. The rate of survival for babies born at the extremes of prematurity (between 22 and 26 weeks) has improved in recent years.

    What is the current rate of overall survival for extreme preterm births?

    A. 25%
    B. 37%
    C. 53%
    D. 63%
    E. 75%

129. Babies born preterm have a much higher risk of suffering from disabilities compared with those born at term.

    What is the most common major long-term consequence of prematurity?

    A. Bronchopulmonary dysplasia
    B. Infective morbidity
    C. Major cerebral scan abnormality
    D. Neurodevelopmental disability
    E. Retinopathy of prematurity

130. The risk of preterm birth is considerably higher in multiple pregnancies than in singleton pregnancies.

    What proportion of twin births take place before 32 weeks of gestation?

    A. 5%
    B. 10%
    C. 15%
    D. 20%
    E. 25%

131. A woman who is 36 weeks pregnant attends the maternity day assessment unit with decreased fetal movements. She has no other symptoms. The CTG and clinical observations are all normal. A dipstick test of a urine sample reveals 1+ proteinuria. The sample is sent for culture and sensitivity. The result is as follows:

    The automated urine microscopy results are:

White blood cells	>100 ($\times 10^6$/l)
Red blood cells	>40–100 ($\times 10^6$/l)
Squamous epithelial cells	≥20 ($\times 10^6$/l)

    The culture results are:

Organism count	10^4–10^5/ml
Organism	Group B *Streptococcus*
Antibiotic sensitivity	Erythromycin, nitrofurantoin, penicillin

    What is the correct management?

    A. No treatment required
    B. Offer IAP only
    C. Send a further specimen and offer IAP if GBS confirmed on a second sample
    D. Treat with erythromycin now and offer IAP
    E. Treat with nitrofurantoin now and offer IAP

132. From which gestational age is cell-free fetal DNA present in reliably measurable levels for aneuploidy screening?

    A. 8 weeks
    B. 10 weeks
    C. 12 weeks
    D. 14 weeks
    E. 16 weeks

133. A woman is found to have an adnexal cyst at her 20-week anomaly scan. What is the most common type of adnexal cystic lesion diagnosed at this gestation?
   A. Corpus luteum cyst
   B. Dermoid cyst
   C. Endometrioma
   D. Fimbrial cyst
   E. Follicular cyst

134. What proportion of terminations of pregnancy in the UK are carried out for fetal abnormality?
   A. 1%
   B. 2%
   C. 5%
   D. 10%
   E. 20%

135. After adjusting for confounding factors, which obstetric factors are associated with partner abuse during pregnancy?

	Postpartum endometritis	Preterm labour	SGA fetus	Urinary tract infection	Vaginal bleeding
A	✓	✓	✓		
B		✓	✓	✓	
C	✓			✓	✓
D	✓		✓		✓
E		✓		✓	✓

EMQs

Options for questions 136–139

A	Amniotic fluid volume and umbilical artery Doppler in 1 week
B	Amniotic fluid volume and umbilical artery Doppler in 2 weeks
C	Amniotic fluid volume and umbilical artery Doppler twice per week
D	Biophysical profile
E	Continue low-risk pathway
F	Ductus venosus Doppler
G	Growth scan in 3–4 weeks
H	Growth scan, amniotic fluid volume
I	Growth scan, amniotic fluid volume and umbilical artery Doppler
J	Growth scan, amniotic fluid volume and umbilical artery Doppler in 2 weeks
K	Middle cerebral artery (MCA) Doppler
L	Serial growth scans from 28 weeks
M	Umbilical vein Doppler
N	Uterine artery Doppler at 18 weeks

For the following clinical scenarios, choose the most important ultrasound scan investigation or action to take next. Assume that you are in a hospital where fetal medicine scanning is available. Each option may be used once, more than once or not at all.

136. A 28-year-old woman has a growth scan as her previous baby was born with a weight below the 5th centile. She is now at 28 weeks of gestation. The growth scan for obstetric history shows that the estimated fetal weight (EFW) is on the 50th centile. Amniotic fluid volume and umbilical artery Doppler are normal.

137. A 32-year-old woman in her first pregnancy is seen at 28 weeks of gestation. She has had a growth scan due to a symphysis fundal height measurement below the 10th centile. The growth scan shows an EFW of <5th centile with normal amniotic fluid volume and umbilical artery Doppler.

138. A 26-year-old patient is seen in the antenatal clinic. She is at 29 + 5 weeks of gestation and has a symphysis fundal height below the 10th centile. She has an ultrasound scan that shows EFW below the 5th centile and a normal amniotic fluid volume with absent end-diastolic flow in the umbilical artery. The CTG is normal.

139. An 18-year-old woman in her first pregnancy has a growth scan at 28 weeks of gestation due to her high BMI of 37 kg/m². The growth scan shows an EFW <10th centile. Amniotic fluid volume is normal and the umbilical artery Doppler shows a raised pulsatility index of >2 standard deviations with end-diastolic flow positive.

Options for questions 140–144

A	Arterial blood gas
B	Compression duplex ultrasound
C	Continue treatment and repeat scan in 7 days
D	Computed tomography pulmonary angiography (CTPA)
E	D-dimer
F	ECG and chest X-ray (CXR)
G	Full blood count (FBC), urea and electrolytes (U&E), liver function test (LFT), coagulation test
H	Magnetic resonance venography
I	Refer back to midwife-led care
J	Start prophylactic low-molecular-weight heparin (LMWH)
K	Start therapeutic dose LMWH
L	Start unfractionated heparin
M	Stop treatment and repeat scan in 3 days
N	Stop treatment and repeat scan in 7 days
O	Thrombophilia screening
P	Ventilation/perfusion (V/Q) scan

For each of the following clinical scenarios, select the most appropriate next step in management from the list of options above. Each option may be used once, more than once or not at all.

140. A 34-year-old patient is seen in the obstetric triage unit out of hours at 26 weeks of gestation with acute pain, tenderness and swelling of her left leg. She is otherwise well with no chest pain or shortness of breath.

141. A 38-year-old patient is seen at 22 weeks of gestation with acute swelling and pain in her right calf. She was started on a therapeutic dose of LMWH and has had a Doppler ultrasound scan that is negative for deep vein thrombosis (DVT). She remains symptomatic.

142. An 18-year-old patient at 35 weeks of gestation has presented with chest pain and shortness of breath. She has a sinus tachycardia and CXR is normal. Laboratory investigations are normal and she has been started on LMWH.

143. A 42-year-old patient is seen at 18 weeks of gestation with chest pain, mild shortness of breath and a swollen left leg. Baseline investigations including bloods, CXR and ECG are normal. She has a duplex ultrasound the same day that confirms left-sided femoral DVT.

144. A 23-year-old patient is referred by the midwife at 38 weeks of gestation with chest pain and shortness of breath. The symptoms resolve but the CTPA scan report states: 'No evidence of embolus in the segmental or subsegmental pulmonary tree, unable to exclude smaller peripheral emboli on CTPA.'

Options for questions 145–148

A	Alternate days
B	At least four times per day
C	Daily
D	Fortnightly
E	Hourly
F	More than four times per day
G	Once only
H	Three times per week
I	Twice per day
J	Twice per week
K	Weekly

For each of the following clinical scenarios, select the single most appropriate frequency to monitor the requested parameter. Each option may be used once, more than once or not at all.

145. A 33-year-old woman is in her first pregnancy at 34 weeks of gestation. She has a blood pressure of 164/108 mmHg that is treated with oral labetalol as an inpatient. Her urinary protein : creatinine ratio is 26 mg/mmol. How often should urinary protein quantification be repeated?

146. A 28-year-old woman is in her first pregnancy at 32 weeks of gestation with a blood pressure of 154/103 mmHg with urinary protein : creatinine ratio of 22 mg/mmol. Treatment with labetalol is commenced. How often should her blood pressure be checked?

147. A 36-year-old woman is in her second pregnancy with dichorionic diamniotic (DCDA) twins at 30 weeks of gestation. Her blood pressure is 153/98 mmHg on two occasions. Her urinary protein : creatinine ratio is 89 mg/mmol. Initial blood tests for FBC, U&E and LFT are normal. How often should these blood tests be repeated?

148. A 29-year-old woman in her first pregnancy has been diagnosed with severe gestational hypertension at 30 weeks of gestation. She has an ultrasound scan that shows a normal growth, amniotic fluid volume and umbilical artery Doppler. How often should the scan be repeated, assuming the growth remains normal and stable?

Options for questions 149–153

A	10 + 0 weeks
B	12 + 0 weeks
C	14 + 0 weeks
D	16 + 0 weeks
E	18 + 0 weeks
F	20 + 0 weeks
G	24 + 0 weeks
H	28 + 0 weeks
I	32 + 0 weeks
J	34 + 0 weeks
K	35 + 0 weeks
L	36 + 0 weeks
M	37 + 0 weeks
N	38 + 0 weeks
O	39 + 0 weeks

For each of the following clinical scenarios pertaining to multiple pregnancy, choose the single most appropriate gestational age from the list above. Each option may be used more than once, more than once or not at all.

149. A 24-year-old woman is referred to the antenatal clinic. She is uncertain of her last menstrual period and is thought to be in the second trimester. An ultrasound scan shows a twin pregnancy. Ideally, by what gestational age should chorionicity have been determined?

150. A 34-year-old woman is found in the first trimester to have an MCDA twin pregnancy. From what gestational age should serial ultrasound scans commence?

151. A 30-year-old woman is found in the first trimester to have a DCDA twin pregnancy. From what gestational age should serial assessment of fetal weight commence?

152. A 25-year-old woman is seen in the antenatal clinic with a DCDA twin pregnancy. It has so far been uncomplicated. From what gestational age should delivery be offered if it remains uncomplicated?

153. A 38-year-old woman is known to have an uncomplicated triplet pregnancy following IVF. From what gestational age should delivery be offered?

Options for questions 154–157

A	Antenatal booking blood tests including hepatitis C screen
B	Antenatal care by consultant obstetrician
C	Clitoral reconstruction
D	Immediate deinfibulation procedure
E	Immediate risk assessment about child safeguarding
F	Inform the police or social services
G	Intrapartum deinfibulation
H	Midwife-led antenatal care
I	Refer to mental health services
J	Refer to safeguarding midwife
K	Review in the presence of a professional interpreter
L	Thorough examination of the genitalia

Each of the following clinical scenarios relates to a woman with FGM in pregnancy. For each patient, select the single most appropriate advice about the next step in management from the list above. Each option may be used once, more than once or not at all.

154. A 22-year-old married British woman of Somali origin attends the consultant antenatal clinic following her routine fetal anomaly scan. She gives a history of having undergone FGM as a young girl at the age of 12 years and suffers from lack of sensation during sexual intercourse. Her 5-year-old son was born via uncomplicated vaginal birth and lives with the woman and her husband.

155. A 19-year-old woman in her first pregnancy is a new arrival in the UK. She attends the early pregnancy unit complaining of lower abdominal pain and vaginal spotting during the past week. There is no bleeding at present. Her home pregnancy test was positive a few weeks ago. She has not yet registered with a GP and does not have a community midwife. A female friend is accompanying her and reveals that the woman had undergone a procedure suggestive of FGM in her early childhood in Africa.

156. A 29-year-old woman in her first pregnancy at 40 weeks of gestation attends the obstetric day assessment unit following a fall onto her abdomen. She has been booked in another hospital and is currently a visitor on holiday in the locality. She gives a history of FGM for which she was to undergo a deinfibulation procedure at 38 weeks of gestation in the hospital where she is booked but was unable to attend. She is not keen on undergoing an examination of her genitalia and wishes to deliver in her own hospital. An abdominal examination and CTG are normal.

157. An obstetric registrar is asked to review a woman in the hospital accident and emergency department with a history of amenorrhoea for 2 months complaining of acute-onset lower abdominal pain. On questioning, she reveals that she was forced to undergo FGM a week ago. Examination reveals a remarkably distended bladder and evidence of freshly healing vulval wounds.

Options for questions 158–160

A	Combined spinal epidural analgesia
B	Inpatient treatment with oral labetalol
C	Intravenous diazepam
D	Intravenous hydralazine
E	Intravenous labetalol infusion
F	Intravenous magnesium sulfate 2–4 g
G	Intravenous magnesium sulfate 2 g loading dose, followed by infusion of 2 g/hour for 24 hours
H	Intravenous magnesium sulfate 4 g loading dose, followed by infusion of 1 g/hour for 24 hours
I	Intravenous phenytoin
J	Oral nifedipine
K	Preload with intravenous 500 ml crystalloid, followed by epidural analgesia
L	Preload with intravenous 500 ml crystalloid, followed by intravenous hydralazine

Each of the following clinical scenarios relates to severe hypertension in pregnancy. For each patient, select the single most appropriate option of management from the list above. Each option may be used once, more than once or not at all.

158. A 32-year-old woman at 37 weeks of gestation has had an eclamptic seizure and is currently receiving treatment with intravenous labetalol. A magnesium sulfate infusion has been running for the last 6 hours. Her blood pressure is 150/100 mmHg, urine output is 200 ml in the last 4 hours and her blood test results are within normal limits. She now has a second eclamptic seizure.

159. A 42-year-old woman has been admitted at 33 weeks of gestation with vomiting and is subsequently found to have severe pre-eclampsia. She is a known asthmatic on treatment with inhaled salbutamol and steroids. Her blood pressure is 170/110 mmHg and urine output is 140 ml in the last 4 hours. Her platelet count is 100×10^9/l. She appears well and her deep tendon reflexes are normal.

160. A 24-year-old woman at 32 weeks of gestation attends the midwife-led antenatal clinic and is found to have a blood pressure of 156/106 mmHg. Urine testing with an automated reagent-strip reader shows proteinuria of 2+ and a spot urinary protein : creatinine ratio of 30 mg/mmol.

Options for questions 161–163

A	Abdominal examination
B	Abdominal ultrasound scan
C	Bimanual vaginal examination
D	CT scan
E	Imaging at 28 weeks of gestation
F	Imaging at 32 weeks of gestation
G	Imaging at 36 weeks of gestation
H	MRI scan
I	Positron emission tomography (PET) scan
J	Speculum examination
K	Transvaginal ultrasound scan
L	Ultrasound scan with colour Doppler
M	Ultrasound scan with power Doppler

For each of the following clinical scenarios, select the single most appropriate management option from the list above. Each option may be used once, more than once or not at all.

161. A 32-year-old woman has her detailed anatomy scan at 20 weeks of gestation. The placenta is situated posteriorly, and it is suspected that the placental edge covers the internal os of the cervix.

162. A 32-year-old woman with a BMI of 35 kg/m² who has had two previous caesarean sections is found to have an anterior placenta at her 20-week scan and further imaging is arranged at 32 weeks of gestation. The findings are similar but the quality of the ultrasound image is poor.

163. A 28-year-old woman in her first pregnancy has a detailed scan at 20 weeks of gestation. This suggests that the placental edge is 1 cm from the internal cervical os. These findings are confirmed by a transvaginal scan. The pregnancy is otherwise uncomplicated.

Options for questions 164–166

A	*Chlamydia trachomatis*
B	Cytomegalovirus
C	Group A *Streptococcus*
D	Group B *Streptococcus*
E	Hepatitis B virus
F	Hepatitis C virus
G	Herpes simplex virus type 1
H	Herpes simplex virus type 2
I	Human immunodeficiency virus (HIV)
J	Human parvovirus B19
K	*Listeria monocytogenes*
L	*Neisseria gonorrhoeae*
M	Rubella virus
N	*Toxoplasma gondii*
O	*Treponema pallidum*
P	Varicella-zoster virus
Q	Zika virus

For each of the following clinical scenarios, select the organism that is the most likely cause of infection from the list above. Each option may be used once, more than once or not at all.

164. A woman experiences low-grade fever in the first trimester of pregnancy but does not seek medical advice. Later during her antenatal care, the fetus is noted to be SGA and is delivered at 38 weeks of gestation following induction of labour. At birth, the infant is noted to be jaundiced with a petechial rash. There is hepatosplenomegaly and microcephaly.

165. A woman who is an asylum seeker in the UK first presents for antenatal care at 36 weeks of gestation. Although it is difficult to determine the precise gestational age, the fetus appears to be small for dates. The woman delivers vaginally at 39 weeks of gestation. The fetus has congenital cataracts and microphthalmia. An echocardiogram shows pulmonary artery stenosis with a patent ductus arteriosus.

166. A British couple visit Cuba for their honeymoon and shortly afterwards the woman finds she is pregnant. For religious beliefs, the couple decline all screening tests. The woman delivers at term. The baby is found to have microcephaly and ventriculomegaly.

Options for questions 167–171

A	Autosomal dominant
B	Autosomal recessive
C	Balanced translocation
D	Maternal non-disjunction
E	Mitochondrial inheritance
F	Mosaicism
G	Paternal non-disjunction
H	Robertsonian translocation
I	Sporadic mutation
J	Triploidy
K	Unbalanced translocation
L	X-linked dominant
M	X-linked recessive
N	Y-linked

For each of the following conditions, give the most common genetic aetiology from the list above. Each option may be used once, more than once or not at all.

167. Down's syndrome

168. Haemophilia A

169. β-Thalassaemia

170. Huntington's disease

171. Duchenne muscular dystrophy

Options for questions 172–175

A	1
B	2
C	3
D	4
E	5
F	6
G	7
H	8
I	10
J	20
K	25
L	30
M	65
N	70
O	100
P	105
Q	110
R	120

For the following patients with antenatal haematological problems, choose the correct value from the list above to answer the question. The required unit is indicated in the question. Each option may be used once, more than once or not at all.

172. A 21-year-old woman is readmitted with an antepartum haemorrhage with a low placenta. She had a recent blood sample sent to the laboratory for group and screen during her last admission. Within how many days should this sample have been sent to be used for the provision of blood?

173. A 22-year-old woman has been found to be anaemic at 28 weeks of gestation. Below what threshold of haemoglobin (in g/l) should supplementation with oral iron be commenced?

174. A 38-year-old woman with β-thalassaemia trait has a haemoglobin level of 95 g/l. Haematinic studies are requested on a sample of her blood. Below what threshold of ferritin (in μg/l) should iron supplementation be commenced?

175. A 28-year-old woman is seen in the antenatal clinic. Her booking blood tests show a normal haemoglobin, but she is found to be iron deficient with a ferritin level of 5 μg /l. What daily dose (in mg) of elemental iron should be prescribed?

Answers

SBAs

96. Answer **C** 3 months

    Explanation
    Conception during tamoxifen therapy should be avoided because of potential teratogenicity, and a 'washout period' of 2–3 months is advised.

    Reference

    RCOG. Pregnancy and breast cancer. *RCOG GTG No. 12*. March 2011.

97. Answer **D** Moderate aerobic exercise for 15 minutes per day three times per week

    Explanation
    Women who have not exercised routinely should begin with 15 minutes of continuous exercise three times weekly, increasing to daily 30-minute sessions.

    Reference

    Kuhrt K, Hezelgrave NL, Shennan AH. Exercise in pregnancy. *The Obstetrician & Gynaecologist* 2015;17:281–7.

98. Answer **E** Head circumference

    Explanation
    Crown–rump length measurement should be used to determine gestational age. If the crown–rump length is >84 mm, the gestational age should be estimated using the head circumference.

    Reference

    NICE. Antenatal care for uncomplicated pregnancies. *NICE Clinical Guideline (CG62)*. Updated January 2017.

99. Answer **B** 800 units

    Explanation
    According to NICE guidelines, this patient has two moderate and one high risk factors for pre-eclampsia and therefore requires 800 units of vitamin D with calcium supplementation. See Table 1 in the reference article.

    Reference

    RCOG. Vitamin D in pregnancy. *RCOG Scientific Impact Paper No. 43*. June 2014.

100. Answer **A** 6 mm

     Explanation
     The presence of an increased nuchal fold (≥6 mm) or two or more soft markers on the routine anomaly scan should prompt the offer of a referral to a fetal medicine specialist or an appropriate healthcare professional with a special interest in fetal medicine.

Reference

NICE. Antenatal care for uncomplicated pregnancies. *NICE Clinical Guideline (CG62)*. Updated January 2017.

101. Answer   **E**   Only when requested by the mother

Explanation
Auscultation of the fetal heart may confirm that the fetus is alive but is unlikely to have any predictive value, and routine listening is therefore not recommended. However, when requested by the mother, auscultation of the fetal heart may provide reassurance.

Reference

NICE. Antenatal care for uncomplicated pregnancies. *NICE Clinical Guideline (CG62)*. Updated January 2017.

102. Answer   **D**   Twice weekly CTG and amniotic fluid volume assessment

Explanation
From 42 weeks, women who decline induction of labour should be offered increased antenatal monitoring consisting of at least twice weekly CTG and ultrasound estimation of maximum amniotic pool depth.

Reference

NICE. Antenatal care for uncomplicated pregnancies. *NICE Clinical Guideline (CG62)*. Updated January 2017.

103. Answer   **D**   Malpresentation at term

Explanation
See Figure 1 in the reference article.

Reference

Dawood R, Altanis E, Ribes-Pastor P, Ashworth F. Pregnancy and spinal cord injury. *The Obstetrician & Gynaecologist* 2014;16:99–107.

104. Answer   **B**   Cognitive behavioural therapy (CBT)

Explanation
For a woman with anxiety disorder in pregnancy or the postnatal period, offer a low-intensity psychological intervention (e.g. facilitated self-help) or a high-intensity psychological intervention (e.g. CBT) as the initial treatment in line with the recommendations set out in the NICE guideline for the specific mental health problem and be aware that:

- Only high-intensity psychological interventions are recommended for PTSD
- High-intensity psychological interventions are recommended for the initial treatment of social anxiety disorder.

Reference

NICE. Antenatal and postnatal mental health: clinical management and service guidance. *NICE Clinical Guideline (CG192)*. Updated August 2017.

105. Answer   C   Postpone the trip if possible

Explanation
A health professional advising a prospective UK resident who is pregnant or thinking about becoming pregnant and who is intending to go to a malaria-endemic area should suggest that the woman considers not going or postponing her trip until she is no longer pregnant.

Reference
RCOG. Prevention of malaria in pregnancy. *RCOG GTG No. 54a.* April 2010.

106. Answer   A   Laser ablation of placental vessels

Explanation
TTTS presenting before 26 weeks of gestation should be treated by fetoscopic laser ablation rather than amnioreduction or septostomy. There is evidence that the fetoscopic laser ablative method should be the Solomon technique.

The conclusion of a Cochrane review was that endoscopic laser coagulation of anastomotic vessels should continue to be considered in the treatment of all stages of TTTS to improve neurodevelopmental outcomes in the child. When compared with amnioreduction, treatment with laser coagulation does not appear to increase or reduce the overall risk of death (stillbirth, neonatal and postneonatal) in this condition, but it appears to result in more children being alive without neurological abnormality.

Amnioreduction can be retained as a treatment option for those situations where the expertise in laser coagulation is not available, pending transfer to a unit where such treatment can be obtained or when the condition is diagnosed after 26 weeks of pregnancy. However, this may complicate future treatment if associated with inadvertent septostomy.

Reference
RCOG. Management of monochorionic twin pregnancy. *RCOG GTG No. 51.* November 2016.

107. Answer   E   Postpone delivery and perform fetal MRI after 4 weeks

Explanation
Clinical management is complex and should be overseen by fetal medicine experts with the knowledge and experience to advise parents about the advantages and disadvantages of different approaches. Rapid delivery is usually unwise, unless at term, as fetal brain injury of the surviving twin occurs at the time of demise of the co-twin. Therefore, immediate delivery only adds prematurity to the possible hypotensive cerebral injury the surviving twin may have already sustained. Serious compromise of the surviving fetus may be anticipated and this should be discussed with parents, including the significant risk of long-term morbidity.

A conservative management policy is often appropriate, with serial fetal brain ultrasound imaging and a fetal cranial MRI scan planned, commonly 4 weeks after the 'sentinel event'. The appearances of intracranial neurological morbidity on ultrasound are variable and may take up to 4 weeks to develop. Fetal MRI provides earlier and more detailed information about brain lesions (haemorrhagic or ischaemic) in the surviving fetus than ultrasound, and its use should be considered.

Reference

RCOG. Management of monochorionic twin pregnancy. *RCOG GTG No. 51*. November 2016.

108. Answer   C   Daily Dopplers and deliver if ductus venosus becomes abnormal

Explanation
In the preterm small-for-gestational-age (SGA) fetus with umbilical artery with absent or reversed end-diastolic velocity (AREDV) detected prior to 32 weeks of gestation, delivery is recommended when ductus venosus Doppler becomes abnormal or umbilical vein pulsations appear, provided the fetus is considered viable and after completion of steroids. Even when venous Doppler is normal, delivery is recommended by 32 weeks of gestation and should be considered between 30 and 32 weeks of gestation.

Unlike conventional CTG, which has high intra- and interobserver variability, cCTG is objective and consistent. Normal ranges for cCTG parameters throughout gestation are available. Fetal heart rate variation is the most useful predictor of fetal well-being in SGA fetuses; an STV of ≤3 ms (within 24 hours of delivery) has been associated with a higher rate of metabolic acidaemia (54.2% versus 10.5%) and early neonatal death (8.3% versus 0.5%).

While cCTG can be used to time delivery where ductus venosus measurement is not available, an STV of ≤3 ms is considered abnormal.

Reference

RCOG. Small-for-gestational-age fetus, investigation and management. *RCOG GTG No. 31*. March 2013.

109. Answer   C   Deinfibulation at 20 weeks

Explanation
For women with type 3 FGM, where adequate vaginal assessment in labour is unlikely to be possible, deinfibulation should be recommended antenatally, usually in the second trimester, typically at around 20 weeks of gestation. Antenatal deinfibulation as an elective procedure ensures that the procedure is performed by an appropriately trained midwife or obstetrician. However, women may prefer deinfibulation during labour, as this is the usual practice in some countries where FGM is prevalent.

Reference

RCOG. Female genital mutilation and its management. *RCOG GTG No. 53*. July 2015.

110. Answer   B   Oligohydramnios

Explanation
A meta-analysis of unexplained antepartum haemorrhage identified ten relevant studies in the previous 38 years, with a limited number of cases; preterm delivery (odds ratio (OR) 3.17, 95% CI 2.76–3.64), stillbirth (OR 2.09, 95% CI 1.43–3.06)

and fetal anomalies (OR 1.42, 95% CI 1.07–1.87) appeared to be increased in frequency.

An epidemiological study of women with unexplained antepartum haemorrhage demonstrated an increased risk of oligohydramnios (OR 6.2, 95% CI 3.1–12.7), prelabour rupture of membranes (OR 3.4, 95% CI 1.8–6.2), fetal growth restriction (OR 5.6, 95% CI 2.5–12.2), preterm labour and caesarean delivery (OR 4.0, 95% CI 2.4–6.6).

Reference

RCOG. Antepartum haemorrhage. *RCOG GTG No. 63.* December 2011.

111. Answer   **E**   Small-for-gestational-age (SGA) fetus

Explanation
In one study, 339 women with a singleton delivery after bariatric surgery (84.4% gastric bypass) were matched to 1277 unexposed women (after adjusting for BMI, parity, age, date of delivery and smoking). Infants in the first group had a shorter mean gestational age (274 versus 278 days), a higher risk of being SGA (adjusted OR (aOR) 2.29, 95% CI 1.32–3.96) and a lower mean birthweight (3312 versus 3585 g), but had a lower risk of being large for gestational age (aOR 0.31, 95% CI 0.15–0.65). When analysing data from women with a gastric bypass alone ($n = $ 286), the risk of SGA was even higher (aOR 2.78, 95% CI 1.56–4.96). With respect to other outcomes, in contrast to smaller studies, no statistically significant differences were found between the groups regarding the risk of gestational diabetes mellitus, pre-eclampsia, labour induction, caesarean section, postpartum haemorrhage, Apgar score <7, admission to the neonatal intensive care unit or perinatal death.

Reference

RCOG. The role of bariatric surgery in improving reproductive health. *RCOG Scientific Impact Paper No. 17.* October 2015.

112. Answer   **D**   1 in 300 pregnancies

Explanation
Risk factors for vasa praevia include placental anomalies such as a bilobed placenta or succenturiate lobes where the fetal vessels run through the membranes joining the separate lobes together, a history of a low-lying placenta in the second trimester, multiple pregnancy and IVF, where the incidence of vasa praevia has been reported to be as high as 1 in 300.

The reasons for this association are not clear, but disturbed orientation of the blastocyst at implantation, vanishing embryos and the increased frequency of placental morphological variations in IVF pregnancies have all been postulated.

Reference

RCOG. Placenta praevia, placenta praevia accreta and vasa praevia: diagnosis and management. *RCOG GTG No. 27.* January 2011.

113. Answer **B** Desquamation of palms and soles

Explanation
Desquamation of the palms and soles is the final (fifth) feature that would confirm the diagnosis. See Appendix 1 in the reference article.

Reference
RCOG. Bacterial sepsis in pregnancy. *RCOG GTG No. 64a*. April 2012.

114. Answer **C** Offer a membrane sweep at 40 weeks onwards

Explanation
Prior to formal induction of labour, women should be offered a vaginal examination for membrane sweeping at the 40- and 41-week antenatal visits for nulliparous women and at the 41-week antenatal visit for parous women.

When a vaginal examination is carried out to assess the cervix, the opportunity should be taken to offer the woman a membrane sweep. Additional membrane sweeping may be offered if labour does not start spontaneously.

Reference
NICE. Induction of labour. *NICE Clinical Guideline (CG70)*. July 2008.

115. Answer **D** 15 weeks

Explanation
Amniocentesis should be performed after 15 (15 + 0) weeks of gestation. Amniocentesis before 14 (14 + 0) weeks of gestation (early amniocentesis) has a higher fetal loss rate and increased incidence of fetal talipes and respiratory morbidity compared with other procedures.

Reference
RCOG. Amniocentesis and chorionic villus sampling. *RCOG GTG No. 8*. June 2010.

116. Answer **B** Speculum examination of vagina

Explanation
In a woman reporting symptoms suggestive of PPROM, offer a speculum examination to look for pooling of amniotic fluid. If pooling of amniotic fluid is observed, do not perform any diagnostic test but offer care consistent with the woman having PPROM. If pooling of amniotic fluid is not observed, consider performing an IGFBP-1 test or PAMG-1 test of vaginal fluid.

Do not use a nitrazine test for diagnosis of PPROM.

Reference
NICE. Preterm labour and birth. *NICE Clinical Guideline (CG25)*. November 2015.

117. Answer **B** Increased observations for 12 hours

Explanation
Term babies who are clinically well at birth and whose mothers have received intrapartum antibiotic prophylaxis (IAP) for prevention of early-onset GBS disease >4 hours before delivery do not require special observation.

How should well babies at risk of early-onset GBS disease whose mothers have not received adequate IAP be monitored? Well babies should be evaluated at birth for clinical indicators of neonatal infection and have their vital signs checked at 0, 1 and 2 hours, and then 2 hourly until 12 hours.

Postnatal antibiotic prophylaxis is not recommended for asymptomatic term infants without known antenatal risk factors.

Reference

RCOG. Early-onset neonatal group B streptococcal disease. *RCOG GTG No. 36*. September 2017.

118. **Answer E** 160 ml one to two times per week

Explanation
If women choose to drink alcohol during pregnancy, they should be advised to drink no more than 1–2 UK units once or twice a week (1 unit equals half a pint of ordinary-strength lager or beer, or one shot (25 ml) of spirits. One small (125 ml) glass of wine is equal to 1.5 UK units). Although there is uncertainty regarding a safe level of alcohol consumption in pregnancy, at this low level there is no evidence of harm to the unborn baby.

Two units of normal-strength wine would equate to approximately 160 ml.

Reference

NICE. Antenatal care for uncomplicated pregnancies. *NICE Clinical Guideline (CG62)*. March 2008.

119. **Answer E** 80%

Explanation
Sensitivity is the ability of an assay under evaluation to identify correctly true positive (reference assay positive) samples. Therefore, sensitivity is the number of true positive samples (A) correctly identified by the assay under evaluation divided by the total number of true positive samples (i.e. those positive by the reference assays $= A + C$), expressed as a percentage, as indicated in the table. It is expressed as: sensitivity $= A/(A + C)$.

	Down's syndrome present	Down's syndrome absent	Total
Test positive	$A = 8$ (true positive)	$B = 4$ (false positive)	12
Test negative	$C = 2$ (false negative)	$D = 86$ (true negative)	88
Total	10	90	100 $A + B + C + D = N$ (total number of tests in study)

Reference

Public Health England. UK Standards for Microbiology Investigations: evaluations, validations and verifications of diagnostic tests. *Public Health England Quality Guidance 1*, Issue 5. June 2014.

120. Answer **E** Angiotensin-converting enzyme (ACE) inhibitors, angiotensin-receptor blockers (ARBs) and thiazides

Explanation
Tell women who take antihypertensive treatments other than ACE inhibitors, ARBs or chlorothiazide that the limited evidence available has not shown an increased risk of congenital malformation with such treatments.

Reference

NICE. Hypertension in pregnancy: diagnosis and management. *NICE Clinical Guideline (CG107)*. Updated January 2011.

121. Answer **B** 125 IU anti-D Ig/ml of fetal red blood cells

Explanation
A dose of 500 IU anti-D Ig intramuscularly is considered sufficient to treat a fetomaternal haemorrhage of up to 4 ml of fetal red blood cells. Where it is necessary to give additional doses of anti-D Ig, as guided by tests for fetomaternal haemorrhage, the dose calculation is traditionally based on 125 IU anti-D Ig/ml of fetal red blood cells for intramuscular administration. However, healthcare professionals should refer to the manufacturer's guidance depending on which product is used.

Reference

Qureshi H, Massey E, Kirwan D, *et al.* BCSH guideline for the use of anti-D immunoglobulin for the prevention of haemolytic disease of the fetus and newborn. *Transfusion Medicine* 2014;24:8–20.

122. Answer **B** Maternal blood test for fetal genotyping for K antigen after 20 weeks of gestation

Explanation
Non-invasive fetal genotyping using maternal blood is now possible for D, C, c, E, e and K antigens. This should be performed in the first instance for the relevant antigen when maternal red blood cell antibodies are present. Genotyping can be undertaken from 16 weeks of gestation for all except K, which can be undertaken from 20 weeks, due to the risk of a false-negative result if performed earlier in pregnancy. Although anti-K titres do not correlate well with either the development or severity of fetal anaemia, titres should nevertheless be measured every 4 weeks up to 28 weeks of gestation and then every 2 weeks until delivery.

Reference

RCOG. Management of red cell antibodies in pregnancy. *RCOG GTG No. 65.* May 2014.

123. **Answer B Combined screening test**

Explanation
Women with monochorionic twins who wish to have aneuploidy screening should be offered nuchal translucency measurements in conjunction with first-trimester serum markers (combined screening test) at 11 + 0 weeks to 13 + 6 weeks of gestation (crown–rump length 45–84 mm).

In women with monochorionic twin pregnancies who 'miss' or who have unsuccessful first-trimester screening for aneuploidy, second-trimester screening by the quadruple test should be offered.

Early data with non-invasive prenatal testing are encouraging, but results should be interpreted with caution until larger studies have been carried out.

Reference
RCOG. Management of monochorionic twin pregnancy. *RCOG GTG No. 51*. November 2016.

124. **Answer A <27 pg**

Explanation
Where prevalence of sickle-cell disease is low (fetal prevalence ≤1.5 cases in 10,000 pregnancies), all pregnant women should be offered screening for haemoglobinopathies using the Family Origin Questionnaire.

If the Family Origin Questionnaire indicates a high risk of sickle-cell disorders, laboratory screening (preferably high-performance liquid chromatography) should be offered.

If the mean corpuscular haemoglobin is <27 pg, laboratory screening (preferably high-performance liquid chromatography) should be offered.

Reference
NICE. Antenatal care for uncomplicated pregnancies. *NICE Clinical Guideline (CG62)*. March 2008.

125. **Answer C To implement postnatal intervention to decrease the risk of mother-to-child transmission.**

Explanation
Serological screening for hepatitis B virus should be offered to pregnant women so that effective postnatal intervention can be offered to infected women to decrease the risk of mother-to-child transmission.

Reference
NICE. Antenatal care for uncomplicated pregnancies. *NICE Clinical Guideline (CG62)*. March 2008.

126. **Answer C 700 µg**

Explanation
The intake of vitamin A during pregnancy should be limited to the recommended daily amount, which, in Europe, is 2310 IU, equivalent to 700 µg. As liver and liver products contain variable and sometimes very high amounts of vitamin A (10,000–38,000 mg per typical portion size of 100 g), these foodstuffs should be

avoided in pregnancy. The consumption of liver and liver products by pregnant women (and particularly the intake of >700 µg) is associated with an increase in the risk of certain congenital malformations.

Reference

NICE. Antenatal care for uncomplicated pregnancies. *NICE Clinical Guideline (CG62)*. March 2008.

127. Answer   **E**   Offer induction of labour immediately and IAP

Explanation
For women undergoing spontaneous rupture of membranes prior to elective caesarean section, IAP for GBS should be offered. The time interval between pregnancies is predictive of recurrent GBS colonisation. Women with GBS colonisation with spontaneous rupture of membranes at term should be offered immediate induction of labour.

Reference

RCOG. Early-onset neonatal group B streptococcal disease. *RCOG GTG No. 36*. September 2017.

128. Answer   **C**   53%

Explanation
Babies born preterm (i.e. before 37 + 0 weeks of pregnancy) have high rates of early, late and postneonatal mortality, with the risk of mortality being inversely proportional to gestational age at birth. Babies who survive have increased rates of disability compared with babies who are not born preterm. Recent UK studies comparing cohorts born in 1995 and 2006 have shown improved rates of survival (from 40% to 53%) for extreme preterm births (born between 22 and 26 weeks).

Reference

NICE. Preterm labour and birth. *NICE Clinical Guideline (CG25)*. November 2015.

129. Answer   **D**   Neurodevelopmental disability

Explanation
The major long-term consequence of prematurity is neurodevelopmental disability. This can range from severe motor abnormalities, such as cerebral palsy, through to less severe cognitive abnormalities.

Reference

NICE. Preterm labour and birth. *NICE Clinical Guideline (CG25)*. November 2015.

130. Answer   **B**   10%

Explanation
The risk of preterm birth is also considerably higher in multiple pregnancies than in singleton pregnancies, occurring in 50% of twin pregnancies (10% of twin births take place before 32 weeks of gestation). The significantly higher preterm delivery rates in twin and triplet pregnancies mean there is increased demand for specialist neonatal resources.

Reference

NICE. Multiple pregnancy: antenatal care for twin and triplet pregnancies. *NICE Clinical Guideline (CG129)*. September 2011.

131. Answer **B** Offer IAP only

Explanation
Clinicians should offer IAP to women with GBS bacteriuria identified during the current pregnancy.

Women with a GBS urinary tract infection (growth of $>10^5$ colony-forming units/ml) during pregnancy should receive appropriate treatment at the time of diagnosis, as well as IAP.

Reference

RCOG. Prevention of early-onset neonatal group B streptococcal disease. *RCOG GTG No. 36*. September 2017.

132. Answer **B** 10 weeks

Explanation
Cell-free fetal DNA is present in reliably measurable levels for aneuploidy screening from 10 weeks of gestation.

Reference

Mackie FL, Allen S, Morris RK, Kilby MD. Cell-free fetal DNA-based noninvasive prenatal testing of aneuploidy. *The Obstetrician & Gynaecologist* 2017;19:211–8.

133. Answer **B** Dermoid cyst

Explanation
Dermoid cysts are the most common adnexal cystic lesions diagnosed after 16 weeks of gestation.

Reference

Alalade AO, Maraj H. Management of adnexal masses in pregnancy. *The Obstetrician & Gynaecologist* 2017;19:317–25.

134. Answer **B** 2%

Explanation
These are classified as ground E abortions (risk that the child would be born 'seriously handicapped'). In England and Wales in 2015, 3213 abortions (2%) were carried out under ground E.

Reference

Department of Health. *Abortion Statistics, England and Wales: 2015*. June 2016.

135. Answer **E** Preterm labour, urinary tract infection and vaginal bleeding

Explanation
After adjusting for confounding factors, studies have demonstrated an association between partner abuse during pregnancy and vaginal bleeding, kidney infections and preterm labour.

Reference

Gottlieb AS. Domestic violence: a clinical guide for women's health care providers. *The Obstetrician & Gynaecologist* 2012;14:197–202.

EMQs

136. Answer **G** Growth scan in 3–4 weeks

137. Answer **J** Growth, amniotic fluid volume and umbilical artery Doppler in 2 weeks

138. Answer **F** Ductus venosus Doppler

139. Answer **C** Amniotic fluid volume and umbilical artery Doppler twice per week

    Explanation
    See Appendix III in the reference article.

Reference

RCOG. The investigation and management of the small-for-gestational-age fetus. *RCOG GTG No. 31*. March 2013.

140. Answer **G** Full blood count (FBC), urea and electrolytes (U&E), liver function test (LFT), coagulation test

    Explanation
    Before anticoagulant therapy is commenced, blood should be taken for a FBC, coagulation screen, U&E and LFT. Performing a thrombophilia screen prior to therapy is not recommended.

141. Answer **M** Stop treatment and repeat scan in 3 days

    Explanation
    If the ultrasound is negative and there is a low level of clinical suspicion, anticoagulant treatment can be discontinued. If the ultrasound is negative and a high level of clinical suspicion exists, anticoagulant treatment should be discontinued but the ultrasound should be repeated on days 3 and 7.

142. Answer **P** Ventilation/perfusion (V/Q) scan

    Explanation
    In women with suspected pulmonary embolism (PE) without symptoms and signs of a DVT, a V/Q lung scan or CTPA should be performed.
    It would be prudent to recommend that lung perfusion scans should be considered the investigation of first choice for young women, especially if there is a family history of breast cancer or the patient has had a previous chest CT scan.

143. Answer   **K**   Start therapeutic dose LMWH

Explanation
In women with suspected PE who also have symptoms and signs of DVT, a compression duplex ultrasound should be performed. If compression ultrasonography confirms the presence of DVT, no further investigation is necessary and treatment for venous thromboembolism (VTE) should commence.

144. Answer   **I**   Refer back to midwife-led care

Explanation
Alternative or repeat testing should be carried out where the V/Q scan or CTPA is normal but the clinical suspicion of PE remains. Anticoagulant treatment should be continued until PE is definitively excluded. The report given with resolved symptoms can be considered normal and therefore treatment can be discontinued.

Reference

RCOG. The acute management of thrombosis and embolism during pregnancy and the puerperium. *RCOG GTG No. 37b.* April 2015.

145. Answer   **C**   Daily

Explanation
For severe gestational hypertension, test for proteinuria daily using an automated reagent-strip reading device or the urinary protein : creatinine ratio.

146. Answer   **J**   Twice per week

Explanation
For moderate hypertension, measure blood pressure at least twice a week.

147. Answer   **H**   Three times per week

Explanation
For moderate pre-eclampsia, carry out blood tests and monitor using the following tests three times per week: kidney function, electrolytes, FBC, transaminases and bilirubin.

148. Answer   **D**   Fortnightly

Explanation
If conservative management of severe gestational hypertension or pre-eclampsia is planned, carry out the following tests at diagnosis:

- Ultrasound fetal growth and amniotic fluid volume assessment
- Umbilical artery Doppler velocimetry.

If the results of all fetal monitoring are normal in women with severe gestational hypertension or pre-eclampsia, do not routinely repeat CTG more than weekly.

In women with severe gestational hypertension or pre-eclampsia, do not routinely repeat ultrasound fetal growth and amniotic fluid volume assessment or umbilical artery Doppler velocimetry more than every 2 weeks.

Reference

NICE. Hypertension in pregnancy: diagnosis and management. *NICE Clinical Guideline (CG107)*. Updated January 2011.

149. Answer **C** 14 + 0 weeks

Explanation
Offer women with twin and triplet pregnancies a first-trimester ultrasound scan when the crown–rump length measures from 45 to 84 mm (at approximately 11 + 0 weeks to 13 + 6 weeks) to estimate gestational age, determine chorionicity and screen for Down's syndrome (ideally, these should all be performed at the same scan).

150. Answer **D** 16 + 0 weeks

Explanation
For MCDA twin pregnancies, combine appointments with scans when the crown–rump length measures from 45 to 84 mm (at approximately 11 + 0 weeks to 13 + 6 weeks) and then at estimated gestations of 16, 18, 20, 22, 24, 28, 32 and 34 weeks.

151. Answer **F** 20 + 0 weeks

Explanation
For DCDA twin pregnancies, combine appointments with scans when the crown–rump length measures from 45 to 84 mm (at approximately 11 + 0 weeks to 13 + 6 weeks) and then at estimated gestations of 20, 24, 28, 32 and 36 weeks. Estimate fetal weight discordance using two or more biometric parameters at each ultrasound scan from 20 weeks.

152. Answer **M** 37 + 0 weeks

Explanation
Offer women with uncomplicated monochorionic twin pregnancies elective birth from 36 + 0 weeks, after a course of antenatal corticosteroids has been offered. For uncomplicated dichorionic twin pregnancies, offer elective birth from 37 + 0 weeks.

153. Answer **K** 35 + 0 weeks

Explanation
Offer women with uncomplicated triplet pregnancies elective birth from 35 + 0 weeks, after a course of antenatal corticosteroids has been offered.

Reference

NICE. Multiple pregnancy: antenatal care for twin and triplet pregnancies. *NICE Clinical Guideline (CG129)*. September 2011.

154. Answer **H** Midwife-led care

Explanation
This woman had an uncomplicated vaginal birth despite having undergone FGM earlier in her childhood. This does not necessarily constitute an indication for high-risk consultant-led care.

If a baby girl is delivered, the safeguarding assessment tool should be filled out and the maternal history of FGM recorded in the child's personal health record ('red book').

155. Answer **L** Thorough examination of the genitalia

Explanation
Any history suggestive of FGM with a history of bleeding in an unbooked woman in her first pregnancy should be an indication to examine her genitalia. Her attendance at the early pregnancy unit should be seen as an opportunity to do that.

156. Answer **G** Intrapartum deinfibulation

Explanation
It is reasonable to carry out deinfibulation in labour. Deinfibulation may be performed antenatally, in the first stage of labour or at the time of delivery, and can usually be performed under local anaesthetic in a delivery suite room. It can also be performed perioperatively after a caesarean section.

157. Answer **D** Immediate deinfibulation procedure

Explanation
This woman appears to have urinary retention secondary to a recent FGM procedure. The priority is to deal with the acute issues. The police and social services must then be informed.

References

RCOG. Female genital mutilation and its management. *RCOG GTG No. 53*. July 2015.
Hussain S, Rymer J. Tackling female genital mutilation in the UK. *The Obstetrician & Gynaecologist* 2017;19:273–8.

158. Answer **F** Intravenous magnesium sulfate 2–4 g

Explanation
Recurrent seizures should be treated with a further dose of 2–4 g given over 5 minutes.

Do not use diazepam, phenytoin or a lytic cocktail as an alternative to magnesium sulfate in women with eclampsia.

159. Answer **L** Preload with intravenous 500 ml crystalloid, followed by intravenous hydralazine

Explanation
Hydralazine is a vasodilator, and its administration must be preceded by an intravenous fluid preload. In this case, magnesium sulfate is not the priority, and in any case, the doses mentioned in the list of options are incorrect. Labetalol is contraindicated, and even if indicated, the preferred method at this level of blood pressure and at this gestational age would be intravenous administration. While nifedipine is also an option in this scenario, the fact she has been vomiting means it would not be the best option.

160. Answer **B** Inpatient treatment with oral labetalol

Explanation
This woman needs admission as she has pre-eclampsia. After admission, a plan for management can be made. None of the other options is appropriate.

Reference

NICE. Hypertension in pregnancy: diagnosis and management. *NICE Clinical Guideline (CG107)*. Updated January 2011.

161. Answer **K** Transvaginal ultrasound scan

Explanation
Transvaginal scans improve the accuracy of placental localisation and are safe, so the suspected diagnosis of placenta praevia at 20 weeks of gestation by abdominal scan should be confirmed by a transvaginal scan.

162. Answer **H** MRI scan

Explanation
Antenatal sonographic imaging can be complemented by MRI in equivocal cases to distinguish those women at special risk of placenta accreta.

163. Answer **F** Imaging at 32 weeks of gestation

Explanation
If the placenta is thought to be low lying (less than 20 mm from the internal os) or praevia (covering the os) at the routine fetal anomaly scan, a follow-up ultrasound examination including a TVS is recommended at 32 weeks of gestation to diagnose a persistent low-lying placenta and/or placenta praevia.

Reference

RCOG. Placenta praevia and placenta accreta: diagnosis and management. *RCOG GTG No. 27a*. September 2018.

164. Answer **B** Cytomegalovirus

Explanation
Cytomegalovirus, a member of the human herpesvirus family, is the most common viral cause of congenital infection, affecting 0.2–2.2% of all live births.

The clinical features of congenital cytomegalovirus at birth include jaundice, petechial rash, hepatosplenomegaly, microcephaly and infants born SGA. Overall, 13% of babies born with congenital cytomegalovirus infection will be symptomatic at birth.

165. Answer **M** Rubella

Explanation
Congenital rubella syndrome involves a wide spectrum of clinical features. In order of decreasing frequency, manifestations include: hearing loss, learning disability, cardiac malformations and ocular defects.

166. Answer **Q** Zika virus

Explanation
Cuba is a high-risk country for Zika virus. The most common congenital anomalies resulting from Zika virus infection include microcephaly, ventriculomegaly and cerebral/ocular calcifications, as well as fetal growth restriction, oligohydramnios and talipes.

References
RCOG. Congenital cytomegalovirus infection: update on treatment. *RCOG Scientific Impact Paper No. 56.* November 2017.
RCOG/RCM/PHE/HPS. Zika virus infection and pregnancy. *Interim RCOG/RCM/PHE/HPS Clinical Guidelines.* Updated July 2017.
To M, Kidd M, Maxwell D. Prenatal diagnosis and management of fetal infections. *The Obstetrician & Gynaecologist* 2009;11:108–16.

167. Answer **D** Maternal non-dysjunction

Explanation
The majority (96%) of Down's syndrome (trisomy 21) arises from non-dysjunction in meiosis. This arises from the maternal cell line in 85% of cases and from the father in 15% of cases. Overall, 2–3% of cases arise from a parental balanced translocation involving chromosome 21 or as a result of a *de novo* translocation. The final 1% are mosaics.

168. Answer **M** X-linked recessive

Explanation
Clinicians should be aware that haemophilia is an X-linked condition associated with the reduction or absence of clotting factor VIII (haemophilia A) or IX (haemophilia B), causing bleeding symptoms.

169. Answer   **B**   Autosomal recessive

Explanation
In theory, genetic counselling for couples who are both carriers of α- or β-thalassaemia is relatively straightforward, in that both conditions are inherited in a simple autosomal-recessive fashion, and fetal testing by chorionic villus sampling, amniocentesis or fetal blood sampling is available.

170. Answer   **A**   Autosomal dominant

Explanation
Huntington's disease is inherited as an autosomal-dominant condition.

171. Answer   **M**   X-linked recessive

Explanation
Duchenne muscular dystrophy is inherited as an X-linked recessive trait and, in the absence of any other family history, the mother of an affected son has a two-thirds risk of being a carrier.

References

Eissa AA, Tuck SM. Sickle cell disease and β-thalassaemia major in pregnancy. *The Obstetrician & Gynaecologist* 2013;15:71–8.
RCOG. Management of inherited bleeding disorders in pregnancy. *RCOG GTG No. 71.* April 2017.
Tobias ES, Connor JM. *Medical Genetics for the MRCOG and Beyond.* Cambridge: Cambridge University Press, 2014.

172. Answer   **C**   3 (days)
Explanation
Group and screen samples used for provision of blood in pregnancy should be <3 days old.

173. Answer   **P**   105 (g/l)

Explanation
Anaemia is defined by a haemoglobin level of <110 g/l in the first trimester, <105 g/l in the second and third trimesters, and <100 g/l in the postpartum period.

174. Answer   **L**   30 (µg/l)

Explanation
Women with known haemoglobinopathy should have serum ferritin checked and be offered oral supplements if their ferritin level is <30 µg/l.

175. Answer **M** 65 (mg)

Explanation

Women with established iron-deficiency anaemia should be given 100–200 mg of elemental iron daily. They should be advised on the correct administration to optimise absorption.

Non-anaemic women identified to be at increased risk of iron deficiency should have their serum ferritin checked early in pregnancy and be offered oral supplements if their ferritin is <30 µg/l.

Non-anaemic iron-deficient women should be offered 65 mg of elemental iron daily, with a repeat haemoglobin and serum ferritin test after 8 weeks.

References

Pavord S, Myers B, Robinson S, *et al.* on behalf of the British Committee for Standards in Haematology. UK guidelines on the management of iron deficiency in pregnancy. *British Journal of Haematology* 2012;156:588–600.

RCOG. Blood transfusion in obstetrics. *RCOG GTG No. 47*. May 2015.

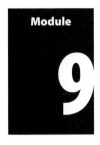

Maternal medicine

SBAs

176. A 26-year-old woman is seen in the combined obstetric cardiology booking clinic at 14 weeks of gestation. She has a history of tetralogy of Fallot that was repaired in childhood.

    What is the main cardiac issue that she potentially faces in pregnancy?

    A. Left ventricular dysfunction
    B. Paradoxical embolism
    C. Profound cyanosis
    D. Pulmonary hypertension
    E. Right ventricular dysfunction

177. A 25-year-old woman is seen in the antenatal clinic at 7 weeks of gestation. She is seen regularly in the congenital heart disease clinic because of Eisenmenger's syndrome secondary to a ventriculoseptal defect.

    What would be the most appropriate advice in terms of management?

    A. Bed rest and home oxygen therapy
    B. Commence oral labetalol
    C. Commence oral sildenafil
    D. Commence thromboprophylaxis with low-molecular-weight heparin (LMWH)
    E. Termination of pregnancy

178. A 28-year-old woman who is currently 12 weeks pregnant has been referred to a breast surgeon after finding a lump in the right breast. Following appropriate imaging and cellular analysis, she is thought to have a stage 1 cancer (no evidence of spread) that is positive for the human epidermal growth factor receptor 2 (HER2) and oestrogen receptor. She declines termination of pregnancy.

    What first-line treatment is most likely to be offered?

    A. Conventional anthracycline chemotherapy
    B. Local radiotherapy with fetal shielding
    C. Primary surgery
    D. Tamoxifen
    E. Trastuzumab

179. A woman presents at 28 weeks of gestation with itching. On examination, she is found to have urticarial-type papules and plaques on her abdomen and thighs. The woman states that she first noticed these lesions in her umbilicus. She also has four 1 cm blisters on her inner thighs. Liver function tests (LFTs) are normal. She is referred to a dermatologist.

     What is the most likely diagnosis?

     A. Atopic eruption of pregnancy
     B. Obstetric cholestasis
     C. Pemphigoid gestationis
     D. Polymorphic eruption of pregnancy
     E. Psoriasis

180. A 36-year-old woman is seen in the booking clinic. She has a history of inflammatory bowel disease and is taking sulfasalazine 4 g/day and folic acid 5 mg/day.

     What is the main fetal risk if she continues this treatment?

     A. Bloody diarrhoea in the newborn
     B. Exomphalos
     C. Intrauterine death
     D. Intrauterine growth restriction
     E. Nephrotoxicity

181. A woman who has sickle-cell disease is seen in the preconception clinic. Her vaccination history is reviewed.

     How often should the pneumococcal vaccine be administered to ensure that she is protected?

     A. Annually
     B. Every 2 years
     C. Every 5 years
     D. Every 10 years
     E. Once only

182. A woman who is 18 weeks pregnant attends a regional tropical diseases clinic with fever, chills and malaise. She has just returned to the UK from working in East Africa. A blood film is examined and a diagnosis of malaria is made. The organism is identified as *Plasmodium vivax*.

     What is the treatment of choice?

     A. Chloroquine
     B. Clindamycin
     C. Mefloquine
     D. Primaquine
     E. Quinine

183. A woman who has previously had genital herpes presents with preterm prelabour rupture of membranes (PPROM) at 32 weeks of gestation. Clinical examination reveals that she has typical lesions of recurrent genital herpes. Assessments of fetal and maternal well-being are otherwise normal.

What is the most appropriate management plan?

	Management of genital herpes	Use of antenatal corticosteroids	Delivery
A	Oral acyclovir	Avoid	Expectant management
B	Oral acyclovir	Usual course	Expectant management
C	Oral acyclovir	Avoid	Expedite with caesarean section
D	Intravenous acyclovir	Usual course	Expedite with caesarean section
E	Intravenous acyclovir	Avoid	Expedite with caesarean section

184. Which two anti-epileptic drugs, when used as low-dose monotherapy, are associated with the lowest risk of congenital malformations?

	Carbamazepine	Lamotrigine	Phenytoin	Pregabalin	Sodium valproate	Topiramate
A	✓	✓				
B			✓			✓
C		✓			✓	
D			✓		✓	
E				✓		✓

185. A woman is screened within a clinical trial and is found to be positive for thyroid peroxidase antibodies but is euthyroid. She opts out of randomisation and becomes pregnant shortly afterwards.

By what factor is she at increased risk of preterm labour compared with women who do not have autoimmune thyroid disease?

A. 1–1.5-fold
B. 2–4-fold
C. 6–8-fold
D. 10–15-fold
E. 20–30-fold

186. A pregnant woman with type 2 diabetes is seeing the diabetes specialist nurse for advice about glucose monitoring in pregnancy.

What would be her target capillary plasma glucose level 2 hours after a meal?

A. 5.3 mmol/l
B. 5.6 mmol/l
C. 6.4 mmol/l
D. 7.2 mmol/l
E. 7.8 mmol/l

187. Which opiate should be avoided as analgesia in labour for pregnant women with epilepsy?

    A. Codeine
    B. Diamorphine
    C. Morphine
    D. Pethidine
    E. Tramadol

188. A 26-year-old woman with epilepsy has just given birth. Her seizures are well controlled with carbamazepine monotherapy. She wishes to have a discussion about postnatal contraception.

    Which hormonal methods of contraception would be considered reliable in this situation?

	Combined hormonal contraceptive	Levonorgestrel-releasing intrauterine system (LNG-IUS)	Medroxyprogesterone acetate (MPA) injection	Progestogen-only pill	Progestogen implant
A	✓	✓			
B		✓	✓		
C			✓	✓	
D				✓	✓
E	✓				✓

189. A 23-year-old woman with β-thalassaemia major attends the antenatal clinic at 8 weeks of gestation. Cardiac function tests performed 12 weeks ago were normal. She has had a splenectomy.

    Her current blood test results are:

Haemoglobin	105 g/l
Platelets	650 × 10⁹/l
Serum fructosamine	275 mmol/l

    What antenatal thromboprophylaxis would be recommended?

    A. Anti-embolic stockings
    B. Aspirin 75 mg daily
    C. Aspirin 75 mg daily plus LMWH
    D. No thromboprophylaxis required
    E. Warfarin

190. A 32-year-old woman with a body mass index (BMI) of 35 kg/m² has just delivered vaginally at term. She is a known carrier of a prothrombin gene mutation.

    For how many days postnatally should she have thromboprophylaxis?

    A. Until mobile
    B. 3 days
    C. 7 days
    D. 10 days
    E. 6 weeks

191. A 33-year-old woman who takes lithium for bipolar disorder is admitted in labour at 39 weeks of gestation. Vaginal examination reveals a fully effaced and 2 cm dilated cervix with intact membranes.

    How should her lithium administration be managed in labour?

    A. Continue treatment with lithium throughout labour
    B. Stop lithium and check plasma levels every 2 hours
    C. Stop lithium and check plasma levels 12 hours after the last dose
    D. Stop lithium and restart after birth
    E. Substitute lithium with a benzodiazepine during labour

192. What are the categories of body weight that require routine measurement of peak anti-Xa activity for women who are under treatment with LMWH for acute venous thromboembolism (VTE) in pregnancy?

	Less than (kg)	More than (kg)
A	45	85
B	50	90
C	55	95
D	60	100
E	65	110

193. What is the incidence of post-thrombotic syndrome (PTS) following a deep venous thrombosis (DVT) in pregnancy?

    A. 32%
    B. 42%
    C. 52%
    D. 62%
    E. 72%

194. A 35-year-old woman is diagnosed with intrahepatic cholestasis of pregnancy and is commenced on therapy with ursodeoxycholic acid (UDCA). Unfortunately, there is no change in either symptoms or biochemical profile.
    Which second-line drug should be considered?

    A. Chlorpheniramine
    B. Cholestyramine
    C. Dexamethasone
    D. Rifampicin
    E. Vitamin K

195. What proportion of pregnancies are affected by gestational hyperthyroidism?

    A. 0.1–0.3%
    B. 0.5–0.7%
    C. 1–3%
    D. 5–7%
    E. 10–30%

196. LFTs may be deranged in 40% of women with hyperemesis gravidarum.
    Which component of LFTs is most frequently abnormal?

    A. Alanine transaminase (ALT)
    B. Alkaline phosphatase
    C. Bile acids
    D. Bilirubin
    E. γ-Glutamyl transferase

197. What is the most common cause of acute kidney injury in pregnancy?

    A. Haemorrhage
    B. Hyperemesis gravidarum
    C. Non-steroidal anti-inflammatory drugs (NSAIDs)
    D. Pre-eclampsia
    E. Urinary retention

198. What proportion of cases of HELLP syndrome will result in an acute kidney injury?

    A. 0.3–1.5%
    B. 3–15%
    C. 23–35%
    D. 43–55%
    E. 63–75%

199. A woman with type 1 diabetes presents at 11 weeks of gestation with diabetic ketoacidosis following several days of vomiting.
    What is the intravenous fluid of choice for initial fluid replacement?

    A. 5% albumin solution
    B. 20% albumin solution
    C. 5% dextrose
    D. Hartmann's solution
    E. 0.9% saline

200. A woman with type 1 diabetes presents with suspected diabetic ketoacidosis (DKA) following a protracted period of vomiting.
    Initial investigations gave the following results:

Serum bicarbonate	13 mmol/l
Serum glucose	18 mmol/l

What would be the threshold value for serum ketones to confirm the diagnosis of DKA?

A. 3 nmol/l
B. 30 nmol/l
C. 300 nmol/l
D. 3 mmol/l
E. 30 mmol/l

EMQs

Options for questions 201–203

A	Magnesium sulfate infusion
B	No treatment required
C	Start amlodipine
D	Start atenolol
E	Start bendroflumethiazide
F	Start chlorothiazide
G	Start hydralazine
H	Start labetalol
I	Start lisinopril
J	Start losartan
K	Start low-dose aspirin
L	Start low-molecular-weight heparin (LMWH)
M	Start vitamins C and E
N	Stop all antihypertensive medication
O	Switch to clopidogrel
P	Switch to enalapril

For each of the following clinical scenarios, choose the single most appropriate pharmacological management from the list of options above. Each option may be chosen once, more than once or not at all.

201. A 39-year-old woman is seen on the postnatal ward just prior to discharge. She had a forceps delivery 2 days earlier. She is planning to continue breastfeeding for at least 6 months. She suffers with chronic hypertension and was taking enalapril prior to pregnancy. Her medication was changed to methyldopa once she had a positive pregnancy test and her blood pressure was stable during pregnancy.

202. A 42-year-old woman with chronic hypertension is seen in the booking clinic at 12 weeks of gestation. She was taking losartan prior to pregnancy and was switched to labetalol once she had a positive pregnancy test at 5 weeks of gestation.

203. A woman is seen in the obstetric day assessment unit at 28 weeks of gestation. She is generally fit and well. She has been referred by her community midwife because her blood pressure is persistently 150/100 mmHg. She has no proteinuria.

Options for questions 204–206

A	Avoidable death
B	Coincidental death
C	Coroner's death
D	Critical death
E	Direct death
F	Early death
G	Fetal death
H	Fortuitous death
I	Indirect death
J	Late death
K	Unavoidable death

For each of the following clinical scenarios, choose the single most appropriate category of death according to the classification by the World Health Organization from the list of options above. Each option may be used once, more than once or not at all.

204. Following an uneventful delivery where the labour was augmented with oxytocin (Syntocinon), a woman suddenly collapses and has a cardiac arrest. Despite appropriate resuscitation, it is not possible to revive her. A post mortem examination records the cause of death as an amniotic fluid embolism.

205. A 25-year-old woman is a poor attender at the antenatal clinic and is known to be a victim of domestic violence. Four weeks after delivery, she is murdered by her ex-partner.

206. A 30-year-old woman with epilepsy that is well controlled with lamotrigine is seen regularly in the antenatal clinic. She fails to follow advice regarding showering rather than bathing. She suffers a seizure while in the bath and drowns.

Options for questions 207–209

A	Carbamazepine
B	Eslicarbazepine
C	Gabapentin
D	Lamotrigine
E	Levetiracetam
F	Oxcarbazepine
G	Phenobarbital
H	Phenytoin
I	Pregabalin
J	Primidone
K	Sodium valproate
L	Tiagabine
M	Topiramate
N	Vigabatrin

For each of the following clinical scenarios, choose the single most appropriate anti-epileptic drug from the list of options above. Each option may be used once, more than once or not at all.

207. A woman taking anti-epileptic medication attends for a routine fetal anomaly scan at 20 weeks of gestation. The fetus is found to have spina bifida and a cleft lip. Which medication is she most likely to be taking?

208. A pregnant woman attends antenatal clinic and is taking a single anti-epileptic drug. She has been informed that the drug she is taking has two main advantages: (1) it carries the lowest risk of congenital malformations; and (2) it does not increase the risk of haemolytic disease of the newborn. Which drug is she most likely to be taking?

209. A woman with epilepsy has a seizure in labour. Benzodiazepines are administered, but the seizures continue. Which second-line therapy should now be administered?

Options for questions 210–212

A	Chlorpropamide
B	Glibenclamide
C	Gliclazide
D	Insulin aspart
E	Insulin detemir
F	Insulin glargine
G	Insulin lispro
H	Isophane insulin (NPH insulin)
I	Metformin
J	No treatment required
K	Phenformin
L	Pioglitazone
M	Rosiglitazone
N	Sitagliptin
O	Tolbutamide
P	Troglitazone

For each of the following clinical scenarios, choose the single most appropriate medication from the list of options above. Each option may be used once, more than once or not at all.

210. A 34-year-old woman is newly diagnosed with gestational diabetes at 24 weeks of gestation. She has modified her diet and undertaken an exercise regime but her plasma glucose levels remain slightly elevated after 2 weeks of this new regime. Which medication is the most appropriate treatment?

211. A woman with type 2 diabetes was taking sitagliptin prior to pregnancy as she could not tolerate the gastrointestinal side effects of metformin. She was switched to insulin therapy in the antenatal period. She has now delivered and wishes to breastfeed. If oral hypoglycaemic agents are required, what treatment would be recommended?

212. A woman with a BMI of 32 kg/m^2 and persistent glycosuria underwent a glucose tolerance test at 24 weeks of gestation.
     Her results are as follows:

Fasting glucose	7.1 mmol/l
2-Hour glucose	10.2 mmol/l

What immediate treatment is recommended?

Options for questions 213–215

A	<50 human immunodeficiency virus (HIV) RNA copies/ml
B	50–399 HIV RNA copies/ml
C	≥400 HIV RNA copies/ml
D	>1000 HIV RNA copies/ml
E	>100,000 HIV RNA copies/ml
F	CD4 cell count <350 cells/μl
G	CD4 cell count ≥350 cells/μl
H	CD4 cell count between 350 and 500 cells/μl
I	CD4 cell count <500 cells/μl
J	CD4 cell count >500 cells/μl
K	Hepatitis B virus (HBV) DNA >2000 IU/ml

For each of the following clinical scenarios, choose the single most applicable test result from the list of options above. Each option may be used once, more than once or not at all.

213. An HIV-positive woman who presented late for antenatal care at 34 weeks of gestation is now in labour. What would be the threshold parameter for offering intrapartum intravenous zidovudine therapy?

214. A 27-year-old woman is reviewed in the antenatal clinic at 36 weeks in her first pregnancy. She has HIV and is on highly active antiretroviral treatment (HAART). What is the threshold parameter for which delivery by elective caesarean section would be recommended?

215. An HIV-positive woman presents with spontaneous rupture of membranes at term. What is the threshold parameter to recommend induction of labour?

Options for questions 216–218

A	Antiphospholipid syndrome
B	Cerebral infarction
C	Cerebral venous thrombosis
D	Drug or alcohol withdrawal
E	Eclampsia
F	Haemorrhagic stroke
G	Hypocalcaemia
H	Hypoglycaemia
I	Hyponatraemia
J	Idiopathic epilepsy
K	Non-epileptic seizure disorder
L	Postdural puncture
M	Secondary epilepsy
N	Thrombotic thrombocytopenic purpura (TTP)

For each of the following clinical scenarios, choose the most likely cause of the convulsion described from the list above. Each option may be used once, more than once or not at all.

216. A 27-year-old woman in her first pregnancy is brought in by ambulance at 37 weeks of gestation having had a seizure. She was visiting her sister and forgot her handheld notes. Her blood pressure is 135/89 mmHg, with a temperature of 37.9°C. A urine dipstick shows 1+ protein and the urine is noted to be very dark. Her blood results are:

Reticulocyte count	High
Platelets	$62 \times 10^9/l$
LFTs	Normal
Creatinine	102 µmol/l
Coagulation	Normal

217. A 23-year-old woman in her first pregnancy is admitted with convulsions, headache and vomiting at 36 weeks of gestation. Her blood pressure is 147/104 mmHg and a urine dipstick shows 2+ proteinuria. Her blood results are:

Haemoglobin	82 g/l
Platelets	$92 \times 10^9/l$
Alanine transaminase	97 IU/l
Creatinine	86 µmol/l

218. A 32-year-old woman in her first pregnancy is admitted after a seizure that lasted 8 minutes. Her antenatal booking notes describe a past history of seizures. On examination, she appears drowsy, with normal reflexes and her plantar reflexes are downgoing. It is somewhat difficult to open her eyes to check her pupils.

Options for questions 219 and 220

A	Biliary cystadenoma
B	Cholangiocarcinoma
C	Focal fatty change
D	Focal nodular hyperplasia
E	Hepatic adenoma
F	Hepatic haemangioma
G	Hepatocellular carcinoma
H	Leiomyoma
I	Lipoma
J	Macroregenerative nodule
K	Mesenchymal hamartoma

The options list contains lesions of the liver occasionally identified during pregnancy. For each of the following clinical scenarios, choose the most likely lesion from the list. Each option may be used once, more than once or not at all.

219. A 25-year-old patient undergoes a liver ultrasound at 28 weeks of gestation for the investigation of epigastric pain. She is found to have a single lesion in the liver measuring 10 cm in diameter.

220. A 29-year-old woman, known to have hepatitis B, undergoes liver screening at 36 weeks of gestation after the finding of abnormal LFTs. She is found to have a lesion of the liver, and on biochemical testing has as an α-fetoprotein level of 1273 ng/ml.

Options for questions 221–223

A	Acute fatty liver of pregnancy
B	Alcoholic liver disease
C	Autoimmune hepatitis
D	Cytomegalovirus hepatitis
E	Epstein–Barr virus hepatitis
F	Haemochromatosis
G	Hepatitis A
H	Hepatitis B
I	Hepatitis C
J	Hepatitis E
K	Hepatocellular carcinoma
L	Intrahepatic cholestasis of pregnancy
M	McArdle's disease
N	Primary biliary cholangitis
O	Primary sclerosing cholangitis
P	Sjögren's syndrome
R	β-Thalassaemia
Q	Wilson's disease

For each of the following clinical scenarios, choose the single most likely cause of liver disease presenting in pregnancy. Each option may be used once, more than once or not at all.

221. A 30-year-old woman in her third pregnancy arrives unbooked from Mumbai at 28 weeks of gestation. She begins to feel unwell at 32 weeks of gestation and develops jaundice, severe fatigue and nausea. She rapidly develops fulminant hepatic failure and encephalopathy. She is transferred to a liver unit, but dies, despite intensive therapy.

222. A 34-year-old woman starts to develop severe pruritus on her limbs and trunk at 34 weeks of gestation. On examination, there is evidence of scratching but no rash. She is afebrile and her urine is dark. LFTs are abnormal with an alanine transaminase (ALT) level of 451 U/l with normal bile acids. Standard liver serological screening is normal.

223. A 23-year-old woman presents with ongoing pruritus that has worsened from 12 weeks of pregnancy.
    Her blood results are:

Albumin	32 g/l
Serum alkaline phosphatase	320 U/l
Serum ALT	35 U/l
Serum bilirubin	20 μmol/l
γ-Glutamyl transferase	40 U/l
Anti-nuclear antibodies	Negative
Anti-mitochondrial antibodies	Positive
Anti-smooth muscle antibodies	Negative
Lupus anticoagulant	Negative

Options for questions 224–226

A	Fasting glucose 4–7 mmol/l, preprandial glucose 5–7 mmol/l
B	Fasting glucose 5–7 mmol/l, preprandial glucose 4–7 mmol/l
C	Fasting glucose ≤5.3 mmol/l, 1-hour postprandial glucose ≤7.8 mmol/l, 2-hour postprandial glucose ≤6.4 mmol/l
D	Fasting glucose ≤5.6 mmol/l, 1-hour postprandial glucose ≤7.2 mmol/l, 2-hour postprandial glucose ≤6.4 mmol/l
E	Fasting glucose >5.6 mmol/l and 2-hour postprandial glucose >7.8 mmol/l
F	Fasting glucose >5.6 mmol/l or 2-hour postprandial glucose >7.8 mmol/l
G	Fasting glucose >6 mmol/l
H	Glucose levels between 4 and 7 mmol/l
I	Glucose levels >4 mmol/l
J	One-hour postprandial glucose 7.8 mmol/l
K	Preprandial glucose 4–6 mmol/l
L	Two-hour postprandial glucose 6.4 mmol/l

Each of the following clinical scenarios relates to a woman with diabetes. From the list of options above, for each woman select the single most appropriate test result. Each option may be used once, more than once or not at all.

224. A 29-year-old diabetic woman is seen in the preconception clinic prior to her first pregnancy. She suffers from type 1 diabetes. She is concerned about the ill effects of diabetes on her baby and asks for advice about the blood glucose levels she should aim for before she gets pregnant.

225. A 32-year-old woman at 32 weeks of gestation is seen in the combined antenatal clinic following a diagnosis of gestational diabetes. What would be the recommendation for target levels of blood glucose during the pregnancy?

226. A 35-year-old woman who had gestational diabetes and gave birth to an infant weighing 4.2 kg has returned to the clinic for a review at 6 weeks postnatal. She has just had a blood test and the result indicates that she will need further testing to see if she has type 2 diabetes.
What test result is she likely to have had?

Options for questions 227–230

A	Anti-embolic stockings only
B	Commence low-molecular-weight heparin (LMWH) in the first trimester and continue for 10 days postpartum
C	Commence LMWH in the first trimester and continue for 6 weeks postpartum
D	Commence LMWH at 28 weeks of gestation and continue for 10 days postpartum
E	Commence LMWH at 28 weeks of gestation and continue for 6 weeks postpartum
F	Commence LMWH at delivery and continue for 10 days postpartum
G	Commence LMWH at delivery and continue for 6 weeks postpartum
H	LMWH at 75% of treatment dose from the first trimester and continue until 6 weeks postpartum
I	Send thrombophilia screen and commence LMWH in the first trimester if positive
J	Short-term LMWH during pro-thrombotic period
K	Thromboprophylaxis not required

Each of the following clinical scenarios relates to thromboprophylaxis in pregnancy. For each patient, select the single most appropriate management from the list above. Each option may be used once, more than once or not at all.

227. A 36-year-old woman, para 3, with a BMI of 32 kg/m² is carrying a twin pregnancy at 11 weeks of gestation and attends the antenatal clinic for advice. She smokes two to five cigarettes a day. Her previous pregnancies were uneventful and resulted in healthy newborn infants at term.

228. A 31-year-old nulliparous woman with a BMI of 29 kg/m² at 26 weeks of gestation asks for advice about thromboprophylaxis because she will be flying to Dubai (a 7-hour flight).

229. A 26-year-old nulliparous woman attends the antenatal clinic at 14 weeks of gestation. Her BMI is 29 kg/m² and she gives a history of previous venous thromboembolism (VTE) during the postoperative recovery period following a hernia operation.

230. A 23-year-old woman with a previous history of unprovoked VTE attends your antenatal clinic at 10 weeks of gestation. She is known to have antithrombin deficiency.

Answers
SBAs

176. Answer **E** Right ventricular dysfunction

Explanation
Women with repaired tetralogy of Fallot usually tolerate pregnancy well; the main issue is right ventricular dysfunction, which can deteriorate in view of the pulmonary regurgitation resulting from earlier surgery.

Reference
Nelson-Piercy C. *Handbook of Obstetric Medicine.* 5th edn. Boca Raton: CRC Press, 2015.

177. Answer **E** Termination of pregnancy

Explanation
Review of the literature between 1997 and 2007 showed maternal death rates of 17% in idiopathic pulmonary arterial hypertension, 28% in congenital heart disease-associated pulmonary hypertension and 33% in other forms. Therefore, such women should be actively advised against pregnancy and adequate contraception recommended, such as the subdermal progestogen-only implant. If they do become pregnant, termination should be offered. Termination itself is associated with maternal mortality in up to 7%, but this is less than that associated with such a pregnancy that is allowed to progress.

Reference
Nelson-Piercy C. *Handbook of Obstetric Medicine.* 5th edn. Boca Raton: CRC Press, 2015.

178. Answer **C** Primary surgery

Explanation
Surgical treatment including locoregional clearance can be undertaken in all trimesters. Breast-conserving surgery or mastectomy can be considered, based on tumour characteristics and breast size, following multidisciplinary team discussion. Reconstruction should be delayed to avoid prolonged anaesthesia and to allow optimal symmetrisation of the breasts after delivery.

Radiotherapy is contraindicated until delivery unless it is lifesaving or to preserve organ function (e.g. spinal cord compression). If necessary, radiotherapy can be considered with fetal shielding or, depending on gestational age, early elective delivery could be discussed. Routine breast/chest wall radiotherapy can be deferred until after delivery.

Systemic chemotherapy is contraindicated in the first trimester because of a high rate of fetal abnormality, but is safe from the second trimester and should be offered according to protocols defined by the risk of breast cancer relapse and mortality.

Tamoxifen and trastuzumab are contraindicated in pregnancy and should not be used.

Reference
RCOG. Pregnancy and breast cancer. *RCOG GTG No. 12.* April 2011.

179. Answer **C** Pemphigoid gestationis

Explanation
Pemphigoid gestationis presents with intense pruritus followed by urticarial papules and plaques, which typically develop on the abdomen and mostly within the umbilical region. Lesions may involve the entire body surface and usually progress to tense blisters. Improvement in late pregnancy is often followed by postpartum flare (75% of cases), after which lesions usually resolve within weeks to months.

Polymorphic eruption of pregnancy starts within the striae distensae on the abdomen, with severely pruritic urticarial papules that coalesce into plaques, spreading to the buttocks and proximal thighs and in severe cases becoming generalised. In contrast to pemphigoid gestationis, the umbilical region is typically spared.

Reference
Vaughan Jones S, Ambros-Rudolph C, Nelson-Piercy C. Skin disease in pregnancy. *British Medical Journal* 2014;348:g3489.

180. Answer **E** Nephrotoxicity

Explanation
Aminosalicylates (sulfasalazine and mesalazine) do not significantly increase the rates of miscarriage, birth defects, low birth weight, stillbirth or preterm delivery, but doses >3 g/day should be avoided because of the risk of fetal nephrotoxicity.

High-dose folic acid supplementation (5 mg/day) is recommended with sulfasalazine use.

Watch for bloody diarrhoea in infants with mesalazine use.

Reference
Kapoor D, Teahon K, Wallace SVF. Inflammatory bowel disease in pregnancy. *The Obstetrician & Gynaecologist* 2016;18:205–12.

181. Answer **C** Every 5 years

Explanation
Women should be given *Haemophilus influenzae* type b and the conjugated meningococcal C vaccine as a single dose if they have not received it as part of primary vaccination. The pneumococcal vaccine (Pneumovax, Sanofi Pasteur MSD Ltd, Maidenhead, UK) should be given every 5 years.

Reference
RCOG. Management of sickle cell disease in pregnancy. *RCOG GTG No. 61*. August 2011.

182. Answer **A** Chloroquine

Explanation
Intravenous artesunate is the treatment of choice for severe *Plasmodium falciparum* malaria. Use intravenous quinine if artesunate is not available. Use quinine and clindamycin to treat uncomplicated *P. falciparum* (or mixed infections, such as *P. falciparum* and *P. vivax*). Use chloroquine to treat *P. vivax*, *P. ovale* or *P. malariae*. Primaquine should not be used in pregnancy

Reference

RCOG. The diagnosis and treatment of malaria in pregnancy. *RCOG GTG No. 54b*. April 2010.

183. Answer **B** Oral acyclovir, usual course of antenatal steroids and expectant management

Explanation
In the case of PPROM before 34 weeks, there is evidence to suggest that expectant management is appropriate, including oral acyclovir 400 mg three times daily for the mother. After this gestation, it is recommended that management is undertaken in accordance with relevant RCOG guidelines on PPROM and antenatal corticosteroid administration to reduce neonatal morbidity and mortality, and is not materially influenced by the presence of recurrent genital herpes lesions.

Reference

BASHH/RCOG. Management of genital herpes in pregnancy. *BASHH/RCOG Guideline*. October 2014.

184. Answer **A** Carbamazepine and lamotrigine

Explanation
In women with epilepsy who are taking anti-epileptic drugs, the risk of major congenital malformation to the fetus is dependent on the type, number and dose of the anti-epileptic drug. Among anti-epileptic drugs, lamotrigine, and carbamazepine monotherapy at lower doses have the least risk of major congenital malformation in the offspring.

Reference

RCOG. Epilepsy in pregnancy. *RCOG GTG No. 68*. June 2016.

185. Answer **B** 2–4-fold

Explanation
Studies have suggested that euthyroid women with autoimmune thyroid disease have a 2–4-fold increased risk of preterm labour.

Reference

Jefferys A, Vanderpump M, Yasmin E. Thyroid dysfunction and reproductive health. *The Obstetrician & Gynaecologist* 2015;17:39–45.

186. Answer   **C**   6.4 mmol/l

    Explanation
    Pregnant women with any form of diabetes should be advised to maintain their capillary plasma glucose below the following target levels if these are achievable without causing problematic hypoglycaemia: fasting: 5.3 mmol/l, and 1 hour after meals: 7.8 mmol/l or 2 hours after meals: 6.4 mmol/l.

    Reference
    NICE. Diabetes in pregnancy: management from preconception to the postnatal period. *NICE Guideline (NG3)*. August 2015.

187. Answer   **D**   Pethidine

    Explanation
    Diamorphine should be used in preference to pethidine for analgesia in labour. Pethidine is metabolised to norpethidine, which is known to be epileptogenic when administered in high doses to patients with normal renal function. Pethidine should therefore be avoided or used with caution. Other methods of analgesia including transcutaneous electrical nerve stimulation (TENS), Entonox and regional analgesia are safe in labour in an epileptic woman.

    Reference
    RCOG. Epilepsy in pregnancy. *RCOG GTG No. 68*. June 2016.

188. Answer   **B**   Levonorgestrel-releasing intrauterine system (LNG-IUS) and medroxyprogesterone acetate (MPA) injection

    Explanation
    Copper intrauterine contraceptive devices (IUCDs), the LNG-IUS and MPA injections should be promoted as reliable methods of contraception that are not affected by enzyme-inducing anti-epileptic drugs.

    Reference
    RCOG. Epilepsy in pregnancy. *RCOG GTG No. 68*. June 2016.

189. Answer   **C**   Aspirin 75 mg daily plus LMWH

    Explanation
    Women with thalassaemia who have undergone splenectomy and have a platelet count above 600×10^9/l should be offered LMWH thromboprophylaxis as well as low-dose aspirin (75 mg/day).

    Reference
    RCOG. Management of beta thalassaemia in pregnancy. *RCOG GTG No. 66*. March 2014.

190. Answer **D** 10 days

Explanation
During the postnatal period, women with two low-risk factors should have thromboprophylaxis for 10 days. Risk factors for this woman are a BMI >30 kg/m² and the prothrombin gene mutation, which is a low-risk thrombophilia.

Reference
RCOG. Reducing the risk of venous thromboembolism during pregnancy and the puerperium. *RCOG GTG No37a*. April 2015.

191. Answer **C** Stop lithium and check plasma levels 12 hours after the last dose

Explanation
Ensure monitoring by the obstetric team when labour starts, including checking plasma lithium levels and fluid balance because of the risk of dehydration and lithium toxicity. Stop lithium during labour and check plasma lithium levels 12 hours after her last dose.

Reference
NICE. Antenatal and postnatal mental health: clinical management and service. *NICE Clinical Guideline (CG192)*. August 2017.

192. Answer **B** Less than 50 kg and more than 90 kg

Explanation
Routine measurement of peak anti-Xa activity for patients on LMWH for treatment of acute VTE in pregnancy or postpartum is not recommended except in women at extremes of body weight (<50 kg and ≥90 kg) or with other complicating factors (e.g. with renal impairment or recurrent VTE).

Reference
RCOG. Thromboembolic disease in pregnancy and the puerperium: acute management. *RCOG GTG No. 37b*. April 2015.

193. Answer **B** 42%

Explanation
PTS is characterised by chronic persistent leg swelling, pain, a feeling of heaviness, dependent cyanosis, telangiectasia, chronic pigmentation, eczema, associated varicose veins and, in the most severe cases, venous ulceration. A case–control study from Norway found a prevalence of PTS of 42% following DVT in pregnancy.

Reference
RCOG. Thromboembolic disease in pregnancy and the puerperium: acute management. *RCOG GTG No. 37b*. April 2015.

194. Answer **D** Rifampicin

Explanation
Given that not all women treated with UDCA have biochemical or symptomatic improvement, a second-line treatment is sometimes considered. Rifampicin is a choleretic antibiotic that has been shown to reduce pruritus and enhance bile acid excretion in primary biliary cirrhosis when used in conjunction with UDCA.

Reference
Geenes V, Williamson C, Chappell LC. Intrahepatic cholestasis of pregnancy. *The Obstetrician & Gynaecologist* 2016;18:273–81.

195. Answer **C** 1–3%

Explanation
Graves' disease is the most common cause of hyperthyroidism in pregnancy, affecting up to 1% of pregnancies. Often, the diagnosis will already have been made, but for those in whom the diagnosis of hyperthyroidism is made in pregnancy, it can be difficult to differentiate from gestational hyperthyroidism, which affects between 1% and 3% of all pregnancies and occurs because of stimulation of thyroid-stimulating hormone receptors by β-human chorionic gonadotropin (β-hCG).

Reference
Jefferys A, Vanderpump M, Yasmin E. Thyroid dysfunction and reproductive health. *The Obstetrician & Gynaecologist* 2015;17:39–45.

196. Answer **A** Alanine transaminase

Explanation
LFTs are abnormal in up to 40% of women with hyperemesis gravidarum, with the most likely abnormality being a rise in transaminases. Bilirubin levels can be slightly raised but without jaundice, and amylase levels can be slightly raised too. These abnormalities improve as the hyperemesis gravidarum resolves.

Reference
RCOG. The management of nausea and vomiting of pregnancy and hyperemesis gravidarum. *RCOG GTG No. 69.* June 2016.

197. Answer **D** Pre-eclampsia

Explanation
Acute kidney injury complicates 1.4% of obstetric admissions in the UK and the most common cause is pre-eclampsia.

Reference
Wiles KS, Banerjee A. Acute kidney injury in pregnancy and the use of non-steroidal anti-inflammatory drugs. *The Obstetrician & Gynaecologist* 2016;18:127–35.

198. Answer **B** 3–15%

Explanation
HELLP syndrome is characterised by **h**aemolysis, **e**levated **l**iver enzymes and a **l**ow **p**latelet count. The incidence of renal impairment is higher in HELLP than in pre-eclampsia, with acute kidney injury complicating 3–15% of cases. The risk of acute kidney injury in HELLP increases if abruption, disseminated intravascular coagulation, sepsis, haemorrhage or intrauterine death occur, and acute kidney injury in the context of HELLP worsens prognosis.

Reference

Wiles KS, Banerjee A. Acute kidney injury in pregnancy and the use of non-steroidal anti-inflammatory drugs. *The Obstetrician & Gynaecologist* 2016;18:127–35.

199. Answer **E** 0.9% saline

Explanation
Fluid replacement should be commenced by infusing isotonic saline (0.9%), as most patients have a negative fluid balance of about 100 ml/kg of body weight. This represents a total fluid deficit of approximately 6–10 l.

Reference

Mohan M, Baagar KAM, Lindow S. Management of diabetic ketoacidosis in pregnancy. *The Obstetrician & Gynaecologist* 2017;19:55–62.

200. Answer **D** 3 mmol/l

Explanation
The Joint British Diabetes Societies Inpatient Care Group guidelines state the following diagnostic criteria for DKA:

- Blood ketone level ≥3.0 mmol/l or urine ketone level >2+
- Blood glucose level >11.0 mmol/l or known diabetes mellitus
- Bicarbonate level <15.0 mmol/l and/or venous pH <7.3.

Reference

Mohan M, Baagar KAM, Lindow S. Management of diabetic ketoacidosis in pregnancy. *The Obstetrician & Gynaecologist* 2017;19:55–62.

EMQs

201. Answer **P** Switch to enalapril

Explanation
If a woman has taken methyldopa to treat chronic hypertension during pregnancy, stop within 2 days of birth and restart the antihypertensive treatment the woman was taking before she planned the pregnancy.

Tell women who still need antihypertensive treatment in the postnatal period that the following antihypertensive drugs have no known adverse effects on babies receiving breast milk: enalapril, labetalol, nifedipine, captopril, atenolol and metoprolol.

202. Answer **K** Start low-dose aspirin

Explanation
Advise women at high risk of pre-eclampsia to take 75 mg of aspirin daily from 12 weeks until the birth of the baby. Women at high risk are those with any of the following:

- Hypertensive disease during a previous pregnancy
- Chronic kidney disease
- Autoimmune disease such as systemic lupus erythematosus or antiphospholipid syndrome
- Type 1 or 2 diabetes
- Chronic hypertension.

203. Answer **H** Start labetalol

Explanation
For the management of pregnancy with moderate gestational hypertension (150/100–159/109 mmHg), treat with oral labetalol as the first-line treatment to keep the diastolic blood pressure between 80 and 100 mmHg and the systolic blood pressure <150 mmHg.

Reference

NICE. Hypertension in pregnancy: diagnosis and management. *NICE Clinical Guideline (CG107)*. Updated January 2011.

204. Answer **E** Direct death

Explanation
The death is a direct result of the pregnancy.

205. Answer **B** Coincidental death

Explanation
The death is not a direct or indirect consequence of the pregnancy.

206. Answer **I** Indirect death

Explanation
The death is related to the pre-existing disease.
   The definitions of pregnancy-related deaths by the World Health Organization (2010) are as follows:

- Maternal: death of a women while pregnant or within 42 days of the end of the pregnancy. This includes death as a result of giving birth, ectopic pregnancy, miscarriage or termination of pregnancy from any cause related to or aggravated by the pregnancy or its management, but not from accidental or incidental causes.
- Direct: deaths resulting from obstetric complications of the pregnant state (pregnancy, labour and puerperium), from interventions, omissions, incorrect treatment, or from a chain of events resulting from any of the above.

- Indirect: deaths resulting from previous existing disease, or disease that developed during pregnancy and which was not the result of direct obstetric causes, but which was aggravated by the physiological effects of pregnancy.
- Late: deaths occurring between 42 days and 1 year after the end of pregnancy (includes giving birth, ectopic pregnancy, miscarriage or termination of pregnancy) that are the result of direct or indirect maternal causes.
- Coincidental: deaths from unrelated causes that happen to occur in pregnancy or the puerperium.

Reference

Knight M, Nair M, Tuffnell D, *et al.* (eds.) on behalf of MBRRACE-UK. *Saving Lives, Improving Mothers' Care: Surveillance of Maternal Deaths in the UK 2012–14 and Lessons Learned to Inform Maternity Care From the UK and Ireland Confidential Enquiries into Maternal Deaths and Morbidity 2009–14*. Oxford: National Perinatal Epidemiology Unit, University of Oxford, 2016.

207. Answer   **K**   Sodium valproate

Explanation
Sodium valproate is associated with neural tube defects, a facial cleft and hypospadias.

208. Answer   **D**   Lamotrigine

Explanation
In women with epilepsy who are taking anti-epileptic drugs (AEDs), the risk of major congenital malformation to the fetus is dependent on the type, number and dose of AEDs. Among AEDs, lamotrigine and carbamazepine monotherapy at lower doses have the lowest risk of major congenital malformation in the offspring.

Enzyme-inducing AEDs (carbamazepine, phenytoin, phenobarbital, primidone, oxcarbazepine, topiramate and eslicarbazepine) are considered to competitively inhibit the precursors of clotting factors and affect fetal microsomal enzymes that degrade vitamin K, thereby increasing the risk of haemorrhagic disease of the newborn.

The drug that fulfils both of these characteristics is therefore lamotrigine.

209. Answer   **H**   Phenytoin

Explanation
If seizures are not controlled, consider administration of phenytoin or fosphenytoin. The loading dose of phenytoin is 10–15 mg/kg by intravenous infusion, with the usual dosage for an adult being about 1000 mg.

Reference

RCOG. Epilepsy in pregnancy. *RCOG GTG No. 68*. June 2016.

210. Answer **I** Metformin

Explanation
Offer metformin to women with gestational diabetes if blood glucose targets are not met using changes in diet and exercise within 1–2 weeks.

211. Answer **B** Glibenclamide

Explanation
Women with pre-existing type 2 diabetes who are breastfeeding can resume or continue to take metformin and glibenclamide immediately after birth, but should avoid other oral blood glucose-lowering agents while breastfeeding.

212. Answer **H** Isophane insulin (NPH insulin)

Explanation
Offer immediate treatment with insulin, with or without metformin, as well as changes in diet and exercise, to women with gestational diabetes who have a fasting plasma glucose level of ≥ 7.0 mmol/l at diagnosis. Isophane insulin is the only short-acting insulin given in the list.

Reference
NICE. Diabetes in pregnancy: management from preconception to the postnatal period. *NICE Guideline (NG3)*. August 2015.

213. Answer **D** >1000 HIV RNA copies/ml

Explanation
Intrapartum intravenous zidovudine infusion is recommended for women with a viral load of >1000 HIV RNA copies/ml of plasma who present in labour or with ruptured membranes, or who are admitted for a planned caesarean section.

214. Answer **C** ≥ 400 HIV RNA copies/ml

Explanation
Where the viral load is ≥ 400 HIV RNA copies/ml at 36 weeks, a planned lower-segment caesarean section is recommended. For a viral load of 50–399 copies/ml, planned lower-segment caesarean section would be offered, and <50 copies/ml vaginal birth would be recommended.

215. Answer **A** <50 HIV RNA copies/ml

Explanation
For the management of spontaneous rupture of membranes:

- If the maternal HIV viral load is <50 HIV RNA copies/ml, immediate induction of labour is recommended, with a low threshold for treatment of intrapartum pyrexia
- If the viral load is >50 HIV RNA copies/ml, then an immediate caesarean section would be offered.

Reference

BHIVA. British HIV Association guidelines for the management of HIV infection in pregnant women 2012 (2014 interim review). *HIV Medicine* 2014;15(Suppl. 4):1–77.

216. Answer   **N**   Thrombotic thrombocytopenic purpura (TTP)

Explanation
The classical pentad of TTP is:

- Microangiopathic haemolytic anaemia
- Thrombocytopenia
- Fever
- Neurological manifestations
- Renal impairment/acute kidney injury.

The clinical features of TTP/haemolytic–uraemic syndrome (HUS) may be confused with pre-eclampsia and particularly HELLP syndrome. However, hypertension is not common in TTP/HUS and there is no coagulopathy. Features include headache, irritability, drowsiness, seizures, coma and fever.

217. Answer   **E**   Eclampsia

Explanation
The features of pre-eclampsia may be mild or delayed.

218. Answer   **K**   Non-epileptic seizure disorder

Explanation
Useful distinguishing features to differentiate a 'psychogenic' non-epileptic seizure from organic non-epileptic seizure or epilepsy include:

- Prolonged/repeated seizures without cyanosis
- Resistance to passive eye opening
- Downgoing plantar reflexes
- Persistence of a positive conjunctival reflex.

Reference

Nelson-Piercy C. *Handbook of Obstetric Medicine*. 5th edn. Boca Raton: CRC Press, 2015.

219. Answer   **F**   Hepatic haemangioma

Explanation
Hepatic haemangiomas are the most common benign tumour of the liver and are present in 2–20% of healthy individuals. They are well-circumscribed lesions that arise from vascular endothelial cells with multiple, large vascular channels supported by collagenous walls. The blood supply arises from the hepatic artery, and the lesion can grow up to 20 cm and cause symptoms.

220.   Answer   **G**   Hepatocellular carcinoma

Explanation

The incidence of hepatocellular carcinoma is increasing in the UK because of cirrhosis linked to obesity and alcohol use. However, the highest rates are found in women from Asian backgrounds with early-onset cirrhosis associated with chronic viral hepatitis B and C. During pregnancy, it has been reported that a serum α-fetoprotein level of >1000 ng/ml can be considered diagnostic; however, this is inconsistent.

Survival appears to be lower in pregnant women, which may be due to the hormonal and immunological influences of pregnancy.

Reference

Milburn J, Black M, Ahmed I, *et al.* Diagnosis and management of liver masses in pregnancy. *The Obstetrician & Gynaecologist* 2016;18:43–51.

221.   Answer   **J**   Hepatitis E

Explanation

Hepatitis E virus is spread by the faecal–oral route and has been associated with drinking contaminated water. The incubation period is 3–8 weeks, with most presenting at 5–6 weeks. The mortality rate is greatly elevated in pregnant women, especially if acquired in the third trimester. While acute fatty liver of pregnancy is a differential, this typically presents later in the third trimester and would be less likely in a multiparous patient.

222.   Answer   **L**   Intrahepatic cholestasis of pregnancy

Explanation

This is a typical presentation of intrahepatic cholestasis of pregnancy. Most cases present in the third trimester. The woman is afebrile, so an infective cause is less likely.

223.   Answer   **N**   Primary biliary cholangitis

Explanation

The ongoing pruritus suggests pre-existing disease. Primary biliary cholangitis may result in worsening pruritus in pregnancy. Alkaline phosphatase and γ-glutamyl transferase levels tend to be raised (although alkaline phosphatase is already raised in pregnancy). The finding of positive anti-mitochondrial antibodies clinches the diagnosis.

Reference

Nelson-Piercy C. *Handbook of Obstetric Medicine.* 5th edn. Boca Raton: CRC Press, 2015.

224. **Answer B** Fasting glucose 5–7 mmol/l, preprandial glucose 4–7 mmol/l

    Explanation
    Advise women with diabetes who are planning to become pregnant to aim for the same capillary plasma glucose target ranges as recommended for all people with type 1 diabetes: a fasting plasma glucose level of 5–7 mmol/l on waking and a plasma glucose level of 4–7 mmol/l before meals at other times of the day.

225. **Answer C** Fasting glucose ≤5.3 mmmol/l, 1-hour postprandial glucose ≤7.8 mmol/l, 2-hour postprandial glucose ≤6.4 mmol/l

    Explanation
    Advise pregnant women with any form of diabetes to maintain their capillary plasma glucose below the following target levels, if these are achievable without causing problematic hypoglycaemia: fasting glucose of 5.3 mmol/l and glucose 1 hour after meals of 7.8 mmol/l or glucose 2 hours after meals of 6.4 mmol/l.

226. **Answer G** Fasting glucose >6 mmol/l

    Explanation
    For women who were diagnosed with gestational diabetes and whose blood glucose levels returned to normal after the birth, offer lifestyle advice (including weight control, diet and exercise) and a fasting plasma glucose test 6–13 weeks after the birth to exclude diabetes (for practical reasons this might take place at the 6-week postnatal check).
        Advise women with a fasting plasma glucose level <6.0 mmol/l that they have a low probability of having diabetes at present and they should continue to follow the lifestyle advice.

    Reference

    NICE. Diabetes in pregnancy: management from preconception to the period. *NICE Guideline (NG3).* Updated August 2015.

227. **Answer C** Commence LMWH in the first trimester and continue for 6 weeks postpartum

    Explanation
    This woman has five antenatal risk factors. Prophylaxis should commence in the first trimester and continue until 6 weeks postpartum.

228. **Answer A** Anti-embolic stockings only

    Explanation
    Any pregnant woman who will be undertaking air travel of >4 hours' duration should be advised to use anti-embolic stockings exerting a calf pressure of 14–15 mmHg.

229. Answer **E** Commence LMWH at 28 weeks of gestation and continue for 6 weeks postpartum

Explanation
In women in whom the original VTE was provoked by major surgery from which they have recovered, and who have no other risk factors, thromboprophylaxis with LMWH can be withheld antenatally until 28 weeks provided no additional risk factors are present (in which case they should be offered LMWH). They require close surveillance for the development of other risk factors.

230. Answer **H** LMWH at 75% of treatment dose from the first trimester and continue until 6 weeks postpartum

Explanation
Women with previous VTE associated with antithrombin deficiency (who will often be on long-term oral anticoagulation) should be offered thromboprophylaxis with higher-dose LMWH (either 50%, 75% or full treatment dose) antenatally and for 6 weeks postpartum or until returned to oral anticoagulant therapy after delivery.

Reference

RCOG. Reducing the risk of venous thromboembolism during pregnancy and the puerperium. *RCOG GTG No37a*. April 2015

Management of labour

SBAs

231. In a 2012 report by the National Health Service Litigation Authority (NHSLA), what was the most common contributor to medicolegal obstetric claims in the UK?

    A. Failure to act
    B. Failure to monitor adequately
    C. Failure to recognise an abnormal cardiotocograph (CTG)
    D. Failure to refer
    E. Inappropriate use of oxytocin (Syntocinon)

232. A 24-year-old woman in her first pregnancy attends for induction of labour at term + 13. She had membrane sweeps at 40 and 41 weeks. She is examined and the cervix is found to be 2 cm dilated and 2 cm long with the fetal head engaged. She does not report any contractions.

    What would be the preferred method of induction of labour?

    A. Amniotomy ± oxytocin (Syntocinon)
    B. Balloon catheter
    C. Membrane sweep
    D. Misoprostol
    E. Vaginal prostaglandin

233. A woman is admitted to the labour ward with intermittent lower abdominal pain and is found to be in preterm labour. Her uterus is contracting three times in 10 minutes and the cervix is 4 cm dilated.

    Until which gestational age should magnesium sulfate be offered?

    A. 29 + 6 weeks
    B. 30 + 6 weeks
    C. 31 + 6 weeks
    D. 32 + 6 weeks
    E. 33 + 6 weeks

234. A 26-year-old woman is seen complaining of regular contractions (one every 10 minutes) at 30 + 3 weeks of gestation. A speculum examination is performed and the cervix appears long but slightly dilated. There is no history of ruptured membranes.

     What investigation should be considered first in this situation?

     A. Fetal fibronectin
     B. Full blood count (FBC) and C-reactive protein (CRP)
     C. No test required – treat as preterm labour
     D. Test for insulin-like growth factor-binding protein-1 (IGFBP-1) or placental α-microglobulin-1 (PAMG-1)
     E. Transvaginal ultrasound

235. While in labour, a woman in her first pregnancy at term is deemed to have an abnormal CTG at 6 cm dilation but is making good progress in labour. Fetal blood sampling (FBS) is performed and the lactate level is 4.9 mmol/l. There was a small acceleration in the fetal heart rate during the process of obtaining the blood sample. The cervix is 7 cm dilated after the FBS.

     What is the recommended management?

     A. Caesarean section
     B. Continue with labour
     C. Repeat the FBS in 30 minutes
     D. Repeat the FBS in 1 hour
     E. Repeat the FBS in 1 hour or sooner if the CTG deteriorates

236. A 30-year-old woman in her first pregnancy is in spontaneous labour and has been using nitrous oxide for analgesia. Vaginal examination a few minutes ago revealed that she is now fully dilated. She has no urge to push.

     What is the most appropriate plan of action?

     A. Advise the woman to start active pushing
     B. Reassess in 1 hour
     C. Reassess in 2 hours
     D. Reassess in 4 hours
     E. Start an oxytocin (Syntocinon) infusion

237. A 41-year-old woman is seen at 36 weeks of gestation. This is her first pregnancy, and a plan for induction of labour at 39 weeks has been made. She is anxious about induction of labour.

     What intrapartum risk is increased for women in this age group who undergo induction of labour compared with expectant management?

     A. Caesarean section
     B. Failed induction of labour
     C. Fetal hypoxia
     D. Instrumental delivery
     E. No additional risk

238. A woman in labour requests an epidural for analgesia, but unfortunately during the siting of the epidural there is inadvertent puncture of the dura mater.
    How likely is it that she will develop a postdural puncture headache?

    A. 5–10%
    B. 15–25%
    C. 30–45%
    D. 70–80%
    E. 100%

239. Concerning the use of FBS to assess fetal acidaemia, what is the main benefit of using lactate alone as opposed to pH?

    A. Improved cord gases at delivery
    B. Improved success rate
    C. Reduced caesarean section rate
    D. Reduced hypoxic ischaemic encephalopathy
    E. Reduced instrumental delivery rate

240. What is the most common cardiac adverse effect associated with the use of atosiban?

    A. Chest pain
    B. Hypotension
    C. Palpitations
    D. Pulmonary oedema
    E. Tachycardia

EMQs

Options for questions 241–244

A	Amniotomy
B	Amniotomy and vacuum extraction of the baby
C	Amniotomy followed by oxytocin (Syntocinon) infusion
D	Assess in 1 hour
E	Assess in 2 hours
F	Assess in 4 hours
G	Deliver by caesarean section
H	Midcavity forceps delivery
I	Oxytocin (Syntocinon) infusion with dose increments every 30 minutes
J	Oxytocin (Syntocinon) infusion with dose increments every 15 minutes
K	Oxytocin (Syntocinon) infusion until there are two to three contractions every 10 minutes

Each of the following clinical scenarios relates to the management of delivery. For each patient, select the single most appropriate management plan from the options above. Each option may be used once, more than once or not at all.

241. A 23-year-old low-risk woman in her first pregnancy is now in established labour following spontaneous rupture of membranes. Vaginal examination at 07:30 hours revealed cephalic presentation and a fully effaced, 4 cm dilated cervix. There are regular uterine contractions of increasing intensity at three to four every 10 minutes. At 11:30 hours, her cervix is 5 cm dilated with the sagittal suture in the transverse position and no further descent of the fetal head. There is no evidence of meconium or caput, and auscultation of the fetal heart is a normal pattern.

242. A 27-year-old woman is in labour for the second time. Clinical findings on vaginal examination are as follows. At 06:30 hours, there is cephalic presentation, and a 4 cm dilated, 0.5 cm long central, soft cervix. At 10:30 hours, there is cervical dilation of 5 cm and a fully effaced cervix and intact membranes. At 12:30 hours, the cervical findings are unchanged, but no membranes are felt.

243. A 32-year-old woman in her first pregnancy at term has been in established labour for 14 hours before a vaginal examination at 12:30 hours finds a fully dilated cervix, clear amniotic fluid, and the fetal head at 0 station and in the right occiput anterior position. At 13:30 hours, she is unable to resist the urge to push and starts voluntary efforts.

244. A 35-year-old woman in her pregnancy at term is in the first stage of labour. She underwent spontaneous rupture of membranes at 19:30 hours. At 21:00 hours, vaginal examination revealed that the cervix was fully effaced and 4 cm dilated. At 01:00 hours, the partogram shows that uterus has been contracting two to three times every 10 minutes and the cervical findings remain the same. The fetal head is at −1 station with the sagittal suture in the transverse position.

Options for questions 245–247

A	Acupuncture
B	Birthing balls and upright posture
C	Codeine
D	Combined spinal–epidural anaesthesia
E	Continuous one-to-one support
F	Diamorphine
G	Epidural anaesthesia
H	Nitrous oxide
I	Paracetamol
J	Pethidine
K	Remifentanil
L	Spinal anaesthesia
M	Transcutaneous electrical nerve stimulation (TENS)
N	Water immersion

For each of the following clinical scenarios, choose the single most appropriate option from the list above. Each option may be used once, more than once or not at all.

245. A 26-year-old woman is being seen in the antenatal clinic with a history of anxiety. She wants to avoid any sort of medication in labour. What single non-invasive measure is likely to provide her with the lowest perception of pain in labour?

246. A 22-year-old woman with a history of epilepsy presents in labour. She has been seizure free for 7 years while not taking any anti-epileptic medications. What method of pain relief should be avoided in this situation?

247. A 27-year-old woman presents in labour at 6 cm dilated. She is a smoker and reports a 1-week history of productive cough and pleuritic-type chest pain. Oxygen saturation is 94% at rest. What labour analgesia in particular should be avoided for this woman?

Options for questions 248–250

A	Abnormal
B	Accelerative
C	Non-reactive
D	Non-reassuring
E	Normal
F	Pathological
G	Reactive
H	Reassuring
I	Sinusoidal
J	Suspicious

For each of the following CTG descriptions, choose the most appropriate overall categorisation of CTG trace. Each description relates to a woman in her first pregnancy in the spontaneous first stage of labour. Each option may be used once, more than once or none at all.

248. The CTG shows a baseline rate of 150 beats per minute (bpm). Accelerations are absent and variability is 7 bpm. There are shallow decelerations occurring with contractions, and the fetal heart rate is falling by 20 bpm from the baseline and lasting 30 seconds, mirroring each contraction for 80 minutes. Contractions are four every 10 minutes. What is the overall classification?

249. The CTG shows a baseline rate of 140 bpm. Accelerations are absent. Variability has been 3 bpm for 25 minutes. There are variable decelerations present, each lasting 70 seconds with every contraction for a duration of 40 minutes, with a delayed recovery and no shouldering. Contractions are three every 10 minutes. How should the decelerations in the CTG trace be described?

250. The CTG shows a baseline rate of 150 bpm and accelerations are present. Baseline variability is 8 bpm, and there are decelerations, with the fetal heart rate dropping by 50 bpm and lasting 70 seconds. The decelerations start following each contraction for the last 25 minutes in a 40-minute trace. Contraction frequency is four every 10 minutes. What is the overall categorisation of the CTG?

Answers
SBAs

231. **Answer   C   Failure to recognise an abnormal cardiotocograph (CTG)**

Explanation
See Figure 5 in the reference article.

Reference
Oláh KSJ, Steer PJ. The use and abuse of oxytocin. *The Obstetrician & Gynaecologist* 2015;17:265–71.

232. **Answer   E   Vaginal prostaglandin**

Explanation
Vaginal prostaglandin E2 (PGE2) is the preferred method of induction of labour, unless there are specific clinical reasons for not using it (in particular, the risk of uterine hyperstimulation). It should be administered as a gel, tablet or controlled-release pessary. Costs may vary over time, and Trusts/units should take this into consideration when prescribing PGE2. For doses, refer to the Summary of Product Characteristics. The recommended regimens are:

- One cycle of vaginal PGE2 tablets or gel: one dose, followed by a second dose after 6 hours if labour is not established (up to a maximum of two doses) or
- One cycle of vaginal PGE2 controlled-release pessary: one dose over 24 hours.

   Amniotomy, alone or with oxytocin (Syntocinon), should not be used as a primary method of induction of labour unless there are specific clinical reasons for not using vaginal PGE2, in particular the risk of uterine hyperstimulation.

Reference
NICE. Inducing labour. *NICE Clinical Guideline (CG70)*. July 2008.

233. **Answer   A   29 + 6 weeks**

Explanation
Intravenous magnesium sulfate should be offered for neuroprotection of the baby to women between 24 weeks and 29 + 6 weeks of pregnancy who are:

- In established preterm labour or
- Having a planned preterm birth within 24 hours.

   Intravenous magnesium sulfate should also be considered for neuroprotection of the baby for women between 30+0 and 33+6 weeks of pregnancy who are:

- In established preterm labour or
- Having a planned preterm birth within 24 hours.

Reference
NICE. Preterm labour and birth. *NICE Guidelines (NG25)*. November 2015.

234. Answer   **E**   Transvaginal ultrasound

Explanation

If the clinical assessment suggests that the woman is in suspected preterm labour and she is 29+6 weeks pregnant or less, advise treatment for preterm labour.

If the clinical assessment suggests that the woman is in suspected preterm labour and she is 30+0 weeks pregnant or more, consider transvaginal ultrasound measurement of cervical length as a diagnostic test to determine the likelihood of birth within 48 hours.

Reference

NICE. Preterm labour and birth. *NICE Guidelines (NG25)*. November 2015.

235. Answer   **A**   Caesarean section

Explanation

Lactate (mmol/l)	pH	Interpretation
≤4.1	≥7.25	Normal
4.2–4.8	7.21–7.24	Borderline
≥4.9	≤7.20	Abnormal

Reference

NICE. Intrapartum care for healthy women and babies. *NICE Clinical Guideline (CG190)*. Updated February 2017.

236. Answer   **B**   Reassess in 1 hour

Explanation

If full dilatation of the cervix has been confirmed in a woman without regional analgesia but she does not get an urge to push, carry out further assessment after 1 hour. Consideration should be given to the use of oxytocin (Syntocinon), with the offer of regional analgesia, for nulliparous women if contractions are inadequate at the onset of the second stage.

Reference

NICE. Intrapartum care for healthy women and babies. *NICE Clinical Guideline (CG190)*. Updated February 2017.

237. Answer   **E**   No additional risk

Explanation

UK data from 2009–10 suggest that if all women aged ≥40 years with a singleton pregnancy had been induced at 39 weeks of gestation instead of at 41 weeks of gestation, 17 stillbirths could have been prevented. This equates to inducing an extra 9350 women, or 550 women to prevent one stillbirth. Inducing at 40 weeks of gestation instead of 41 weeks would prevent seven stillbirths and require an extra 4750 women to be induced.

In a study by Walker *et al.* (2016), a total of 619 women aged ≥35 years underwent randomisation with respect to induction of labour or expectant management. In an intention-to-treat analysis, there were no significant between-group differences in the percentage of women who underwent a caesarean section (98 of 304 women in the induction group (32%) and 103 of 314 women in the expectant-management group (33%); relative risk 0.99, 95% confidence interval (CI) 0.87–1.14) or in the percentage of women who had a vaginal delivery with the use of forceps or vacuum (115 of 304 women (38%) and 104 of 314 women (33%), respectively; relative risk 1.30, 95% CI 0.96–1.77). There were no maternal or infant deaths and no significant between-group differences in the women's experience of childbirth or in the frequency of adverse maternal or neonatal outcomes.

References
RCOG. Induction of labour at term in older mothers. *RCOG Scientific Impact Paper No. 34.* February 2013.

Walker KF, Bugg GJ, Macpherson M, *et al.* Randomized trial of labor induction in women 35 years of age or older. *New England Journal of Medicine* 2016;374:813–22.

238. **Answer D 70–80%**

Explanation
See Box 2 in the reference article.

Reference
Revell K, Morrish P. Headaches in pregnancy. *The Obstetrician & Gynaecologist* 2014;16:179–84.

239. **Answer B Improved success rate**

Explanation
A Cochrane meta-analysis compared analysis of lactate and pH in fetal scalp blood during labour and found no differences in fetal/neonatal outcome or operative interventions but a significantly higher success rate with lactate compared with pH (risk ratio 1.10; 95% CI 1.08–1.12). Only two trials were included in this meta-analysis, and approximately 90% of the cases were from one randomised controlled trial. However, in a recently published large observational study, where the above clinical guidelines were used, the FBS frequency was 11%, and out of these 9% were acidaemic (>4.8 mmol/l). This implies that only 1% of all deliveries had an FBS lactate indicating operative/instrumental delivery.

Reference
RCOG. Is it time for UK obstetricians to accept fetal scalp lactate as an alternative to scalp pH? *RCOG Scientific Impact Paper 47.* January 2015.

240. **Answer E Tachycardia**

Explanation
Atosiban has a better maternal cardiac adverse effect profile than β-mimetics in terms of tachycardia (5.5% versus 75.5%), chest pain (1.1% versus 4.8%) and palpitations (2.2% versus 15.6%). Pulmonary oedema occurred in two women in the β-mimetic group.

Reference

Groom KM, Bennett PR. Tocolysis for the treatment of preterm labour – a clinically based review. *The Obstetrician & Gynaecologist* 2004;6:1.

EMQs

241. Answer   **E**   Assess in 2 hours

242. Answer   **I**   Oxytocin (Syntocinon) infusion with dose increments every 30 minutes

243. Answer   **D**   Assess in 1 hour

244. Answer   **I**   Oxytocin (Syntocinon) infusion with dose increments every 30 minutes

Explanation
If a delay in the established first stage is suspected, assess all aspects of progress in labour when diagnosing delay, including:

- Cervical dilation of <2 cm in 4 hours for first labours
- Cervical dilation of <2 cm in 4 hours or a slowing in the progress of labour for second or subsequent labours.

Whether or not a woman has agreed to an amniotomy, advise all women with suspected delay in the established first stage of labour to have a vaginal examination 2 hours later, and diagnose delay if progress is <1 cm.

If oxytocin is used, ensure that the time between increments of the dose is no more frequent than every 30 minutes. Increase oxytocin until there are four to five contractions every 10 minutes.

For a nulliparous woman, suspect delay if progress (in terms of rotation and/or descent of the presenting part) is inadequate after 1 hour of active second stage. Offer a vaginal examination and then offer amniotomy if the membranes are intact.

For a multiparous woman, suspect delay if progress (in terms of rotation and/or descent of the presenting part) is inadequate after 30 minutes of active second stage. Offer a vaginal examination and then offer amniotomy if the membranes are intact.

References

NICE. Intrapartum care for healthy women and babies. *NICE Clinical Guideline (CG190)*. Updated February 2017.
RCOG. Operative vaginal delivery. *RCOG GTG No. 26*. January 2011.

245. Answer   **E**   Continuous one-to-one support

Explanation
Evidence suggests that pain perception is strongly influenced by the attitude and behaviour of the woman's caregiver, which is probably the single most important factor in a woman's perception of pain during labour and childbirth.

246. Answer   J   Pethidine

Explanation
Diamorphine should be used in preference to pethidine for analgesia in labour. Pethidine is metabolised to norpethidine, which is known to be epileptogenic when administered in high doses to patients with normal renal function. Pethidine should therefore be avoided or used with caution.

247. Answer   K   Remifentanil

Explanation
Widespread national and international implementation has been hampered by concerns over the safety of remifentanil patient-controlled analgesia (PCA). Respiratory depression is reported in up to 32% of patients and 5% encounter oxygen saturations <90%. In a UK survey, 11% of respondents reported critical incidences relating to the use of remifentanil and respiratory depression.

   A comprehensive list of relative contraindications to remifentanil PCA is yet to be established but could include morbid obesity, clinical features of a chest infection and women in their first pregnancy who are at risk of prolonged labour.

References
Alleemudder DI, Kuponiyi Y, Kuponiyi C, *et al*. Analgesia for labour: an evidence based insight for the obstetrician. *The Obstetrician & Gynaecologist* 2015;17:147–55.
RCOG. Epilepsy in pregnancy. *RCOG GTG No. 68*. June 2016.

248. Answer   E   Normal

Explanation
The description given is of early decelerations, which can be considered normal in an otherwise normal CTG.

249. Answer   A   Abnormal

Explanation
Variable decelerations with any concerning characteristics in >50% of contractions for 30 minutes (or less if there are any maternal or fetal clinical risk factors) would be classed as an abnormal feature.

250. Answer   J   Suspicious

Explanation
This describes late decelerations, which would be classified as non-reassuring up to 30 minutes and abnormal after 30 minutes. One non-reassuring feature would make the overall classification suspicious.

Reference
NICE. Intrapartum care for healthy women and babies. *NICE Clinical Guideline (CG190)*. Updated February 2017.

SBAs

251. A woman delivered her first baby spontaneously 40 minutes ago and had oxytocin (Syntocinon) 10 IU intramuscularly for active management of the third stage of labour. The placenta has still not delivered, with no signs of separation. She is not bleeding, has intravenous access *in situ* and is haemodynamically stable.

    What would be the appropriate action?

    A. Manual removal of the placenta
    B. Oxytocin (Syntocinon) 20 IU in 20 ml of saline into the umbilical vein
    C. Oxytocin (Syntocinon) 40 IU intravenous infusion at 125 ml/hour
    D. Oxytocin (Syntocinon) 5 IU intravenously
    E. Oxytocin/ergometrine 5 IU/500 µg (Syntometrine) intramuscularly

252. A 31-year-old woman presents in preterm labour at 34 weeks of gestation. Her labour progresses quickly and she delivers a baby boy. Both mother and baby appear to be in good health, and the woman requests delayed cord clamping.

    What time frame would be recommended for delayed cord clamping in this situation?

    A. 10–30 seconds
    B. 30 seconds–3 minutes
    C. 4–6 minutes
    D. 6–10 minutes
    E. Do not recommend delayed cord clamping

253. A woman in the first stage of labour is diagnosed with inadequate progress. The CTG trace is classified as suspicious, and a plan is made to conduct a category 2 caesarean section.

    Within how many minutes from the decision should the baby be delivered?

    A. 30 minutes
    B. 45 minutes
    C. 60 minutes
    D. 75 minutes
    E. 90 minutes

254. A woman has been pushing in the second stage of labour for 2 hours. The head is two-fifths palpable abdominally, at −1 station, with caput and moulding. A decision is taken to proceed to delivery by caesarean section.
   Which complication is more likely for this woman when compared with a caesarean section in the first stage of labour?
   A. Bladder injury
   B. Blood loss >1000 ml
   C. Intraoperative uterine trauma
   D. Perinatal asphyxia
   E. Venous thromboembolism

255. What is the recommended uterotonic regime for routine management of the third stage at caesarean section?
   A. Oxytocin (Syntocinon) 10 IU intravenously
   B. Oxytocin (Syntocinon) 5 IU intravenously
   C. Oxytocin (Syntocinon) 5 IU intravenously with 40 IU oxytocin infusion
   D. Oxytocin/ergometrine 5 IU/500 µg (Syntometrine) intramuscularly
   E. Oxytocin/ergometrine 5 IU/500 µg (Syntometrine) with 40 IU oxytocin (Syntocinon) infusion

256. What is the most common reason for litigation following a shoulder dystocia?
   A. Birth asphyxia
   B. Brachial plexus injury
   C. Clavicular fracture
   D. Humeral fracture
   E. Maternal trauma

257. What proportion of women who are planning a vaginal breech birth will require an emergency caesarean section?
   A. 10%
   B. 20%
   C. 30%
   D. 40%
   E. 50%

258. For women with a breech presentation after 39 weeks of gestation, how many times higher is the perinatal mortality rate associated with a planned vaginal breech birth compared with an elective caesarean section?
   A. Two times
   B. Three times
   C. Four times
   D. Five times
   E. Ten times

259. What is the single best predictor of a successful vaginal birth after a caesarean section?

A. Gestation when in labour
B. History of a previous vaginal birth
C. Maternal age
D. Scar thickness measured by ultrasound
E. Type of caesarean section

260. Following a prolonged second stage of labour, a woman is taken to theatre for a trial of forceps delivery. Examination in theatre reveals the fetal head to be one-fifth palpable per abdomen. On vaginal examination, the station of the fetal head is +1.
How would the forceps delivery be classified?

A. High
B. Unclassifiable
C. Low
D. Mid
E. Outlet

EMQs

Options for questions 261–265

A	Attach fetal scalp electrode
B	Delivery by caesarean section
C	Digital examination of the vagina and cervix
D	Fetal scalp blood sampling
E	Induction of labour
F	Intermittent auscultation of the fetal heartbeat
G	Magnesium sulfate infusion
H	Nifedipine for tocolysis
I	Nitrazine test
J	Rescue cervical cerclage
K	Ritodrine infusion
L	Test for insulin-like growth factor-binding protein-1 (IGFBP-1)
M	Ultrasound scan

Each of the following clinical scenarios relates to management of delivery. For each clinical scenario, select the single most appropriate management option from the list above. Each option may be used once, more than once or not at all.

261. A 45-year-old woman, a mother of two children, has been admitted with symptoms suggestive of preterm rupture of membranes 12 hours ago at 29 weeks of gestation. She complains of intermittent abdominal pain. A sterile speculum examination of the vagina is inconclusive because of laxity of the vaginal wall, which obscures the view of the cervix. There is no obvious collection or pooling of amniotic fluid in the vagina. The uterus appears irritable and the fetus is in cephalic presentation.

262. A 28-year-old woman in her third pregnancy at 32 + 3 weeks of gestation is in labour following the spontaneous onset of uterine contractions 2 days ago. A vaginal examination reveals intact forewaters, and a fully effaced and 7 cm dilated cervix with the fetal head at 0 station. Her body mass index (BMI) is 32 kg/m^2 and the CTG has been reassuring since admission. In the last hour, it has become difficult to interpret the CTG because of difficulty in monitoring the fetal heartbeat due to many episodes of loss of contact.

263. A woman in her first pregnancy is admitted to the labour ward with severe pre-eclampsia at 29 weeks of gestation. She has commenced treatment with intravenous labetalol. Her uterine contraction frequency is about three every 10 minutes and the fetus is in cephalic presentation with the fetal head three-fifths palpable abdominally. A vaginal examination reveals a fully effaced and 4 cm dilated cervix.

264. A 35-year-old woman with a history of recurrent miscarriage and no living children was admitted to the ward a week ago with symptoms of threatened preterm labour at 26 weeks of gestation. She was treated with tocolytics, and prophylactic steroids were administered. She is now at 27 + 3 weeks of gestation and is very anxious because of the prospects of poor prognosis following a preterm birth. There has been no uterine activity over the last 5 days. A vaginal speculum examination reveals intact membranes and a 50% effaced cervix dilated to 5 cm. A vaginal swab taken a week ago has shown no growth of any pathological microbes.

265. A 28-year-old woman, the mother of three children, presents with symptoms of threatened preterm labour at 30 weeks of gestation. She gives a history of a previous preterm birth at 32 weeks of gestation. Following a speculum examination, the fetal fibronectin concentration is found to be 50 ng/ml. A transvaginal ultrasound scan reveals the cervical length to be 15 mm.

Options for questions 266–268

A	Delivery of the posterior arm
B	Downward traction following delivery of the head
C	Kiwi delivery
D	Manual rotation of the fetal head
E	Primary caesarean section
F	Rotational forceps
G	Rubin maneouvre
H	Traction forceps in occipitoanterior position
I	Traction forceps in occipitoposterior position
J	Vaginal breech delivery
K	Vaginal disimpaction of the fetal head
L	Ventouse delivery

For each of the following childbirth-related complications, choose the single most likely method of delivery or manoeuvre associated with that complication. Each option may be used once, more than once or not at all.

266. Subgaleal haematoma.

267. Obstetric anal sphincter injuries (OASIS).

268. Reversion to malposition.

Options for questions 269–270

A	Carbetocin
B	Carboprost (Hemabate)
C	Ergometrine
D	Misoprostol
E	Oxytocin (Syntocinon) 5 IU intramuscularly
F	Oxytocin (Syntocinon) 10 IU intramuscularly
G	Oxytocin (Syntocinon) 5 IU intravenous injection
H	Oxytocin (Syntocinon) 10 IU intravenous injection
I	Oxytocin (Syntocinon) infusion
J	Oxytocin/ergometrine (Syntometrine)
K	Physiological third stage
L	Uterine massage

From the list of options above, choose the most appropriate uterotonic agent for each of the following clinical scenarios? Each option may be used once, more than once or not at all.

269. A low-risk woman in her first pregnancy has an uncomplicated labour and delivers by spontaneous vaginal delivery.

270. A woman with gestational diabetes, but no other medical problems, has just delivered twins. Twin 1 was delivered by forceps due to a delay in the second stage of labour. Twin 2 delivered spontaneously.

Answers
SBAs

251. Answer   **A**   Manual removal of the placenta

Explanation
With respect to a retained placenta:

- Do not use umbilical vein agents if the placenta is retained
- Do not use intravenous oxytocic agents routinely to deliver a retained placenta
- Give intravenous oxytocic agents if the placenta is retained and the woman is bleeding excessively.

If the placenta is retained and there is concern about the woman's condition:

- Offer a vaginal examination to assess the need to undertake manual removal of the placenta
- Explain that this assessment can be painful and advise her to have analgesia.

Do not carry out uterine exploration or manual removal of the placenta without an anaesthetic.

Reference

NICE. Intrapartum care for healthy women and babies. *NICE Clinical Guideline (CG190)*. Updated February 2017.

252. Answer   **B**   30 seconds–3 minutes

Explanation
If a preterm baby (born vaginally or by caesarean section) needs to be moved away from the mother for resuscitation, or there is significant maternal bleeding:

- Consider milking the cord and
- Clamp the cord as soon as possible.

Wait at least 30 seconds, but no longer than 3 minutes, before clamping the cord of preterm babies if the mother and baby are stable. Position the baby at or below the level of the placenta before clamping the cord.

Reference

NICE. Preterm labour and birth. *NICE Guideline (NG25)*. November 2015.

253. Answer   **D**   75 minutes

Explanation
Perform a category 2 caesarean section in most situations within 75 minutes of making the decision.

Reference

NICE. Caesarean section. *NICE Clinical Guideline (CG132)*. August 2012.

254. Answer **B** Blood loss >1000 ml

Explanation
In the referenced study, compared with caesarean section in the first stage of labour, women undergoing caesarean section at the second stage were 4.6 times more likely to have composite intraoperative complications (95% confidence interval (CI) 2.7–7.9, *P* < 0.001), 3.1 times more likely to have blood loss >1000 ml (95% CI 1.3–7.4, *P* = 0.01), and 2.9 times more likely to have complications of intraoperative trauma (relative risk 2.6, *P* < 0.001) and infants with perinatal asphyxia (relative risk 1.5, *P* < 0.05).

Reference
Tempest N, Navaratnam K, Hapangama DK. Management of delivery when malposition of the fetal head complicates the second stage of labour. *The Obstetrician & Gynaecologist* 2015;17:273–80.

255. Answer **B** Oxytocin (Syntocinon) 5 IU intravenously

Explanation
Oxytocin 5 IU by slow intravenous injection should be used during caesarean section to encourage contraction of the uterus and decrease blood loss.

Reference
NICE. Caesarean section. *NICE Clinical Guideline (CG132)*. August 2012.

256. Answer **B** Brachial plexus injury

Explanation
Neonatal brachial plexus injury is the most common cause for litigation related to shoulder dystocia and is the third most litigated obstetric-related complication in the UK.

Reference
RCOG. Shoulder dystocia. *RCOG GTG No. 42*. March 2012.

257. Answer **D** 40%

Explanation
Women should be informed that maternal complications are least with successful vaginal birth; a planned caesarean section carries a higher risk, but the risk is highest with emergency caesarean section, which is needed in approximately 40% of women planning a vaginal breech birth.

Reference
RCOG. Management of breech presentation. *RCOG GTG No. 20b*. March 2017.

258. Answer   C   Four times

    Explanation
    Women should be informed that when planning delivery for a breech baby, the risk of perinatal mortality is approximately 0.5 in 1000 with caesarean section after 39 + 0 weeks of gestation and approximately 2.0 in 1000 with a planned vaginal breech birth.

    Reference
    RCOG. Management of breech presentation. *RCOG GTG No. 20b*. March 2017.

259. Answer   B   History of a previous vaginal birth

    Explanation
    Women with one or more previous vaginal births should be informed that a previous vaginal delivery, particularly previous vaginal birth after a caesarean (VBAC), is the single best predictor of successful VBAC and is associated with a planned VBAC success rate of 85–90%.

    Reference
    RCOG. Birth after previous caesarean birth. *RCOG GTG No. 45*. October 2015.

260. Answer   D   Mid

    Explanation
    For operative vaginal delivery, the classification of a midcavity forceps delivery is when the fetal head is no more than one-fifth palpable per abdomen.
        The leading point of the skull is above station plus 2 cm but not above the ischial spines.

    Reference
    RCOG. Operative vaginal delivery. *RCOG GTG No. 26*. February 2011.

EMQs

261. Answer   L   Test for insulin-like growth factor-binding protein-1 (IGFBP-1)

    Explanation
    A test for IGFBP-1 has a high sensitivity and specificity for detection of PROM. Digital examination risks the introduction of infection. It is important to know about PROM before making any further management plans.

262. Answer   F   Intermittent auscultation of the fetal heartbeat

    Explanation
    Intermittent auscultation is an option for fetal monitoring in established preterm labour.

263. Answer **G** Magnesium sulfate infusion

Explanation
The magnesium sulfate is for neuroprotection as the woman seems to be in established preterm labour but is going to take a few hours before she delivers.

264. Answer **J** Rescue cervical cerclage

Explanation
With this history, it will be worth taking the small risk associated with rescue cerclage. The uterus is relaxed and there is no evidence of infection.

265. Answer **H** Nifedipine for tocolysis

Explanation
The fibronectin test is negative and the cervical length is short, although it is not <15 mm. However, her history of a previous preterm birth is the greatest risk factor and she should be offered treatment with nifedipine.

References

NICE. Preterm labour and birth. *NICE Guidelines (NG25)*. November 2015.
RCOG. The investigation and management of the small-for-gestational age fetus. *RCOG GTG No. 31*. March 2013.

266. Answer **L** Ventouse delivery

Explanation
Although the ventouse has been popular for managing fetal malposition in recent years, it is associated with a significantly higher risk of failure (22.4% versus 3.7% for Kielland forceps) and increased admissions to the neonatal unit (12.1% versus 10.3% for Kielland forceps). Scalp lacerations and cephalohaematoma are common, and subaponeurotic, subgaleal and intracranial haemorrhage also occur.

267. Answer **F** Rotational forceps

Explanation
Of all operative vaginal delivery methods, Kielland forceps are associated with the highest risk of OASIS. However, it has been demonstrated that this risk can be mitigated and OASIS rates kept lower than national UK level 5 with high levels of training and supervision. Kielland forceps require advanced operator skills, including both decision-making and technical components. If those requirements are fulfilled, Kielland forceps are likely to be the most effective method to manage malposition of the fetal head in the second stage of labour and reduce primary emergency caesarean section and emergency caesarean section for failed rotational ventouse.

268. Answer **D** Manual rotation of the fetal head

Explanation
Problems associated with this method in particular include the baby rotating back to a malposition between manual rotation and forceps or ventouse being applied, resulting in potential inaccurate positioning of the forceps/ventouse and the risk of cord prolapse following disimpaction of the head, leading to an obstetric emergency.

Reference

Tempest N, Navaratnam K, Hapangama DK. Management of delivery when malposition of the fetal head complicates the second stage of labour. *The Obstetrician & Gynaecologist* 2015;17:273–80.

269. Answer **F** Oxytocin (Syntocinon) 10 IU intramuscularly

Explanation
For women without risk factors for postpartum haemorrhage delivering vaginally, oxytocin (10 IU by intramuscular injection) is the agent of choice for prophylaxis in the third stage of labour. A higher dose of oxytocin is unlikely to be beneficial.

270. Answer **J** Oxytocin/ergometrine (Syntometrine)

Explanation
Oxytocin/ergometrine may be used in the absence of hypertension in women at increased risk of haemorrhage as it reduces the risk of minor postpartum haemorrhage (500–1000 ml of blood).

Reference

RCOG. Prevention and management of postpartum haemorrhage. *RCOG GTG No. 52.* December 2016

Postpartum problems

SBAs

271. Regarding postpartum family planning, when is the soonest after delivery that a copper intrauterine contraceptive device (IUCD) can be inserted?

    A. Immediately after the third stage of labour is complete
    B. Just prior to leaving the labour ward/delivery room
    C. Just prior to discharge from hospital
    D. 1 week postnatally
    E. 6 weeks postnatally

272. According to the published literature, what is the only obstetric factor that is consistently associated with an increased risk of postpartum psychosis?

    A. Male infant
    B. Maternal age >45 years
    C. Premature delivery
    D. Primiparity
    E. Ventouse delivery

273. Following an episiotomy repair under local anaesthetic, a midwife requests a prescription for a non-steroidal anti-inflammatory drug (NSAID) for ongoing analgesia. Which NSAID carries the greatest risk of the development of acute renal failure?

    A. Diclofenac
    B. Ibuprofen
    C. Indomethacin
    D. Naproxen
    E. Paracetamol

274. A woman who was delivered at 35 weeks of gestation due to pre-eclampsia has ongoing hypertension requiring treatment postpartum. The woman suffers with asthma but has never been hospitalised.
    What would be the most appropriate antihypertensive agent?

    A. Atenolol
    B. Bendroflumethiazide
    C. Enalapril
    D. Labetalol
    E. Nifedipine

275. During a massive postpartum haemorrhage, a woman is found to have a fibrinogen level of 1.5 g/l.

What is the most appropriate product to elevate her fibrinogen levels?

A. Cryoprecipitate
B. Fibrinogen concentrate
C. Fresh frozen plasma
D. Tranexamic acid
E. Whole blood

276. Following delivery, when is the peak in the absolute risk of venous thromboembolism?

A. 1–3 weeks
B. 4–6 weeks
C. 6–12 weeks
D. 3–6 months
E. 6–12 months

277. Methyldopa is often discontinued in the postnatal period due to its association with postnatal depression.

What other side effects are often found with this medication in the postpartum period?

	Postural hypotension	Flushing	Renal impairment	Cough	Sedation
A	✓	✓			
B		✓	✓		
C	✓			✓	
D		✓			✓
E	✓				✓

278. A 25-year-old woman who previously used the combined oral contraceptive pill (COCP) has just delivered and has requested contraceptive advice prior to discharge from hospital. She is fit and well. She has decided not to breastfeed.

At what point in the postpartum period could she restart the COCP?

A. Immediately
B. 1 week
C. 3 weeks
D. 6 weeks
E. 6 months

279. A 38-year-old woman has had her first baby by caesarean section 7 days ago. She is seen by her community midwife and appears to be low in mood with reduced appetite and is sent to hospital for review. There is no suicidal ideation or thoughts to harm her baby, and she is diagnosed with mild depression. The woman's case notes indicate that her mother suffered from bipolar disorder and committed suicide.

What would be the most appropriate action?

A. Admit for observation
B. Commence fluoxetine
C. Discharge to GP
D. Offer counselling
E. Refer to perinatal mental health services

280. Following an eclamptic fit, a woman who is 2 days postpartum develops an aspiration pneumonia and, despite intensive care treatment, dies.

How would this maternal death be classified according to World Health Organization (WHO) criteria?

A. Coincidental
B. Direct
C. Fortuitous
D. Indirect
E. Late

EMQs

Options for questions 281–283

A	Cerebral tumour
B	Cerebral venous sinus thrombosis
C	Dural puncture headache
D	Idiopathic intracranial hypertension
E	Meningitis
F	Migraine
G	Posterior reversible encephalopathy syndrome
H	Pre-eclampsia
I	Reversible cerebral vasoconstriction syndrome (RCVS)
J	Simple headache
K	Sinusitis
L	Subarachnoid haemorrhage
M	Tension headache

For each of the following clinical descriptions of headaches in the postpartum period, select the most likely cause from the list of options above. Each option may be used once, more than once or not at all.

281. A 23-year-old woman with a body mass index (BMI) of 45 kg/m^2 is now 36 hours postemergency caesarean section for failure to progress in labour. She is complaining of a frontal headache that developed over the last few hours. The headache is worse every time she stands up to care for her baby. A neurological examination and ophthalmic fundoscopy are both normal.

282. A 33-year-old woman with a BMI of 32 kg/m^2 is 4 days postnormal vaginal delivery on the midwife-led unit. She complains of a pulsating left-sided headache that has developed over the last 30 minutes. She is nauseous and has vomited twice, and is asking to lie still in a darkened room. Observations are normal, and a neurological examination and ophthalmic fundoscopy are normal.

283. A 31-year-old woman, now 14 days postdelivery, presents for the fourth time postpartum with a sudden-onset headache, like being hit over the head, associated with vomiting, an aversion to light and blurred vision. She had a CT scan after the first episode that was normal.

Options for questions 284–286

A	Amoxicillin
B	Benzylpenicillin
C	Cefuroxime
D	Clarithromycin
E	Clindamycin
F	Co-amoxiclav
G	Erythromycin
H	Gentamicin
I	Meropenem
J	Metronidazole
K	Piperacillin
L	Vancomycin

For each of the following clinical scenarios, select the single most appropriate choice of antibiotic based on the information provided. Each option may be chosen once, more than once or not at all.

284. A 26-year-old woman is diagnosed with severe pyelonephritis 2 days after a caesarean section. Culture of a midstream urine sample grows an extended-spectrum β-lactamase (ESBL)-producing organism. She has no known allergies, and is given a single dose of gentamicin. What antibiotic should also be commenced?

285. A 24-year-old woman is 6 days postpartum. She complains of having had a sore throat for the last 2 days, and culture of a throat swab has confirmed the presence of group A *Streptococcus*. It is suspected that she is developing toxic shock syndrome. Which antibiotic should be used in order to switch off exotoxin production?

286. A 32-year-old woman develops sepsis 2 days after a caesarean section. She is a nurse and is known to carry methicillin-resistant *Staphylococcus aureus* (MRSA). Which antibiotic should be used to ensure that MRSA is treated effectively?

Options for questions 287–290

A	Alcohol withdrawal
B	Amphetamine overdose
C	Baby blues
D	Bipolar disorder
E	Borderline personality disorder
F	Depression
G	Early-onset severe panic disorder
H	Generalised anxiety disorder
I	Obsessive compulsive disorder
J	Postnatal depression
K	Postpartum confusional state
L	Puerperal psychosis
M	Schizophrenia

For each of the following clinical scenarios, choose the single most appropriate diagnosis from the list of options above. Each option may be chosen once, more than once or not at all.

287. A 23-year-old woman is seen 4 days postnatally in obstetric triage after self-presenting after cutting her wrists at 03:00 hours. There is no ongoing bleeding from her injuries. She reports that she had got upset as her boyfriend had been out and came home late. They are now joking with each other and appear very affectionate.

288. A 31-year-old woman is 3 days postdelivery and presents with anxiety. She appears very frightened and exhibits paranoid ideation that her family is trying to take her baby away. She has a history of schizophrenia but has been stable without treatment for 5 years.

289. A 40-year-old woman is 2 weeks postnatal after her first pregnancy. She had a caesarean section and she has no past medical or mental health history. She has not been sleeping, and has been feeling very low and crying a lot. The baby has been readmitted due to excessive weight loss.

290. A 24-year-old woman has delivered her first baby by caesarean section. She is seen by the midwife 3 days postpartum with emotional instability, insomnia and agitation. She seems to improve a little over the following 72 hours but continues to have similar symptoms intermittently over the next 6 weeks. The baby is well looked after.

Answers
SBAs

271. Answer   **A**   Immediately after the third stage of labour is complete

Explanation
IUCDs can be inserted following expulsion of the placenta. It is most convenient and best practice to insert them immediately after the placenta has been delivered.

Reference
RCOG. Best practice in postpartum family planning. *RCOG Best Practice Paper 1.* June 2015.

272. Answer   **D**   Primiparity

Explanation
An increased risk of postpartum psychosis has been reported with a number of obstetric factors including: primiparity, pregnancy and delivery complications, delivery by caesarean section, having a female baby and a shorter gestation period. However, findings are consistent only for primiparity.

Reference
Di Florio A, Smith S, Jones I. Postpartum psychosis. *The Obstetrician & Gynaecologist* 2013;15:145–50.

273. Answer   **D**   Naproxen

Explanation
Comparative data regarding the most 'renal-friendly' NSAIDs are limited. Naproxen has been shown to carry the highest risk of acute renal failure. Indomethacin has been associated with more nephrotoxicity than other NSAIDs in terms of nephritis and hyperkalaemia, and fenoprofen has been associated with the highest risk of nephrosis.

Reference
Wiles KS, Banerjee A. Acute kidney injury in pregnancy and the use of non-steroidal anti-inflammatory drugs. *The Obstetrician & Gynaecologist* 2016;18:127–35.

274. Answer   **E**   Nifedipine

Explanation
A suggested regimen might be labetalol (provided there is no history of asthma) with second- and third-line agents of calcium antagonist and an angiotensin-converting-enzyme (ACE) inhibitor (such as enalapril), respectively.

Reference
Smith M, Waugh J, Nelson-Piercy C. Management of postpartum hypertension. *The Obstetrician & Gynaecologist* 2013;15:45–50

275. Answer   **A**   Cryoprecipitate

Explanation
Cryoprecipitate should be used for fibrinogen replacement.
   The appropriate fibrinogen intervention trigger or target level is unknown. A pragmatic view based on available evidence is that, during continuing postpartum haemorrhage, cryoprecipitate or fibrinogen concentrate should be used to maintain a fibrinogen level of at least 2 g/l, even if the prothrombin time (PT) or activated partial thromboplastin time (aPTT) is normal. Fibrinogen loss can be replaced by cryoprecipitate or fibrinogen concentrate, although fibrinogen concentrate is not licensed for acquired hypofibrinogenaemia in the UK.

Reference
RCOG. Prevention and management of postpartum haemorrhage. *RCOG GTG No. 52.* December 2016.

276. Answer   **A**   1–3 weeks

Explanation
The relative risk postpartum is 5-fold higher compared with antepartum, and a systematic review of the risk of postpartum venous thromboembolism (VTE) found that the risk varied from 21- to 84-fold from the baseline non-pregnant, non-postpartum state in studies that included an internal reference group. The absolute risk peaked in the first 3 weeks postpartum (421 per 100,000 person-years; 22-fold increase in risk).

Reference
RCOG. Reducing the risk of venous thromboembolism during pregnancy and the puerperium. *RCOG GTG No. 37a.* April 2015.

277. Answer   **E**   Postural hypotension and sedation

Explanation
While methyldopa remains a safe option for treatment of hypertension in the postnatal period, particularly in women who have had good antenatal control with the agent, most authorities advise that it should be discontinued because of its maternal side effects, in particular sedation, postural hypotension and postnatal depression.

Reference
Smith M, Waugh J, Nelson-Piercy C. Management of postpartum hypertension. *The Obstetrician & Gynaecologist* 2013;15:45–50.

278. Answer   **C**   3 weeks

Explanation
Women who are not breastfeeding may start the COCP at 3 weeks postpartum unless they have additional risk factors for VTE, in which case they should not start the COCP until 6 weeks after childbirth.

Reference
RCOG. Best practice in postpartum family planning. *RCOG Best Practice Paper No. 1.* June 2015.

279. Answer   E   Refer to perinatal mental health services

Explanation
The good practice guidelines developed by the RCOG suggest that the following scenarios are indications for referral to specialised perinatal mental health services where available, or otherwise to general psychiatry services:

- Current severe psychiatric symptoms
- A history of serious postpartum illness, bipolar disorder or schizophrenia
- On complex psychotropic medication schemes.

Moreover, the guidelines suggest that referral should be considered for those with moderate symptoms developed in late pregnancy or early postpartum, or with mild symptoms and a family history of bipolar disorder or puerperal psychosis.

Reference

Di Florio A, Smith S, Jones I. Postpartum psychosis. *The Obstetrician & Gynaecologist* 2013;15:145–50.

280. Answer   **B**   Direct

Explanation
Direct maternal deaths are classified as deaths resulting from obstetric complications of the pregnant state (pregnancy, labour and puerperium), from interventions, omissions, incorrect treatment, or from a chain of events resulting from any of the above.

Reference

Knight M, Nair M, Tuffnell D, *et al.* (eds.) on behalf of MBRRACE-UK. *Saving Lives, Improving Mothers' Care: Surveillance of Maternal Deaths in the UK 2012–14 and Lessons Learned to Inform Maternity Care From the UK and Ireland Confidential Enquiries into Maternal Deaths and Morbidity 2009–14*. Oxford: National Perinatal Epidemiology Unit, University of Oxford, 2016.

EMQs

281. Answer   **C**   Dural puncture headache

Explanation
Puncture of the dura occurs in 0.5–2.5% of epidurals. If accidental dural puncture occurs with an epidural needle, there is a 70–80% chance of a postdural puncture headache. The headache is usually in the fronto-occipital regions and radiates to the neck; it is characteristically worse on standing and typically develops 24–48 hours postpuncture.

Conservative management includes hydration and simple analgesics. Untreated, the headache typically lasts for 7–10 days but can last up to 6 weeks. An epidural blood patch has a 60–90% cure rate.

282. Answer   **F**   Migraine

Explanation
A migraine is classically:

- Unilateral
- Pulsating
- Builds up over minutes to hours
- Moderate to severe in intensity
- Associated with nausea and/or vomiting and/or sensitivity to light and/or sensitivity to sound
- Disabling
- Aggravated by routine physical activity.

Migraine is classified by the presence or absence of aura. Pregnancy can alter migraine with aura and trigger attacks of aura without headache as a result of high plasma concentrations of oestrogen.

283. Answer   **I**   Reversible cerebral vasoconstriction syndrome (RCVS)

Explanation
RCVS is a cerebrovascular disorder associated with multifocal arterial constriction and dilation. It has a significant association with the postpartum period. RCVS is characterised by recurrent sudden-onset and severe headaches over 1–3 weeks, often accompanied by nausea, vomiting, photophobia, confusion and blurred vision. Diagnosis requires the demonstration of diffuse arterial beading on cerebral angiography with resolution within 1–3 months. It is in the differential of a postpartum thunderclap headache often made after subarachnoid haemorrhage has been excluded but the headaches recur.

Reference
Morrish P. Headaches in pregnancy. *The Obstetrician & Gynaecologist* 2014;16:179–84.

284. Answer   **I**   Meropenem

Explanation
Treat acute pyelonephritis with gentamicin and meropenem.

285. Answer   **E**   Clindamycin

Explanation
Clindamycin is not nephrotoxic and switches off the production of superantigens and other exotoxins.

286. Answer   **L**   Vancomycin

Explanation
MRSA may be resistant to clindamycin; hence, if the woman is or is highly likely to be MRSA-positive, a glycopeptide such as vancomycin or teicoplanin may be added until sensitivity is known.

Reference
RCOG. Bacterial sepsis following pregnancy. *RCOG GTG No. 64b*. April 2012.

287. Answer   E   Borderline personality disorder

Explanation
Borderline personality disorder is characterised by significant instability of interpersonal relationships, self-image and mood, and impulsive behaviour. There is a pattern of sometimes rapid fluctuation from periods of confidence to despair, with fear of abandonment and rejection, and a strong tendency towards suicidal thinking and self-harm. Transient psychotic symptoms, including brief delusions and hallucinations, may also be present. It is also associated with substantial impairment of social, psychological and occupational functioning and quality of life. People with borderline personality disorder are particularly at risk of suicide.

288. Answer   L   Puerperal psychosis

Explanation
Puerperal psychosis is, by definition, a psychotic illness that arises in a previously well woman within a defined period after childbirth. The term covers those women who have a lifetime first-onset psychotic illness following childbirth. It also covers women who have previously had a psychotic illness but have been well in the years preceding their pregnancy.

289. Answer   J   Postnatal depression

Explanation
Severe postnatal depressive illness has an early onset in the first few weeks following birth, but, unlike puerperal psychosis, this tends to be gradual and does not clearly manifest until 4–6 weeks postpartum or later.

The core symptoms are the same as depressive illness at other times. These include the so-called 'biological syndrome', now referred to as the 'somatic subtype', of early morning wakening, diurnal variation of mood, slowing of mental functioning, impaired concentration, and overvalued ideas of incompetence and guilt. These are often accompanied by loss of appetite and weight, loss of spontaneity and enjoyment (anhedonia) and difficulty in coping with the tasks of everyday life.

The baby has been readmitted, suggesting that day-to-day life and care of the newborn has been affected.

290. Answer   C   Baby blues

Explanation
The 'blues' affect 50–80% of all new mothers. This condition is self-limiting and lasts for approximately 48 hours, but it can recur periodically over the next 6–8 weeks, particularly when the mother is very tired.

References

NICE. Borderline personality disorder: recognition and management. *NICE Clinical Guideline (CG78)*. January 2009.
Oates M. Postnatal affective disorders. Part 1: an introduction. *The Obstetrician & Gynaecologist* 2008;10:145–50.

SBAs

291. A 52-year-old woman with a body mass index (BMI) of 32 kg/m² presents with irregular vaginal bleeding. An ultrasound scan demonstrates a thickened endometrium, and an endometrial biopsy confirms endometrial hyperplasia without atypia. A levonorgestrel-releasing intrauterine system (LNG-IUS) is inserted.

     What follow-up should be arranged?

     A. Annual endometrial biopsies for life
     B. Endometrial biopsy at 3 and 6 months and discharge if normal
     C. Endometrial biopsy at 6 and 12 months and discharge if normal
     D. Endometrial biopsy at 6 and 12 months and then annually for life
     E. No follow-up required once the LNG-IUS is inserted

292. During an MRI scan for back pain, a 68-year-old woman was found to have an incidental finding of a 4 cm simple ovarian cyst. This was confirmed by a transvaginal ultrasound scan. She had a hysterectomy at the age of 38 years for heavy menstrual bleeding but her ovaries were conserved. Her serum CA125 level was 17 IU/l.

     What is the most appropriate management?

     A. Arrange a follow-up ultrasound scan in 4 months
     B. Laparotomy and bilateral salpingo-oophorectomy
     C. Perform an ultrasound-guided aspiration
     D. Reassure and discharge
     E. Refer to multidisciplinary team meeting

293. A healthy 40-year-old woman presents to the gynaecology clinic with heavy menstrual bleeding. History, examination and an ultrasound scan suggest the presence of adenomyosis, but no other pathology.

     What would be considered the first-line treatment?

     A. Cyclical oral progestogens
     B. Endometrial ablation
     C. Insertion of an LNG-IUS
     D. Total abdominal hysterectomy
     E. Total laparoscopic hysterectomy

294. A 35-year-old woman presents to the gynaecology clinic with heavy menstrual bleeding and opts to have an LNG-IUS inserted. She is warned of the possibility of changes to her bleeding pattern.

    For how long should she be advised to persevere with any unwanted changes to her bleeding pattern in order to see the maximum benefits of treatment?

    A. Three cycles
    B. Six cycles
    C. Nine cycles
    D. 12 cycles
    E. No specified time

295. What is the most common subtype of vulval lichen planus to cause vulval symptoms?

    A. Classical
    B. Erosive
    C. Hypertrophic
    D. Hypotrophic hyperpigmented
    E. Non-classical

296. What are the three most prevalent symptoms in women with peritoneal endometriosis?

	Chronic pelvic pain	Cyclical intestinal complaints	Deep dyspareunia	Dysmenorrhoea	Heavy menstrual bleeding	Infertility
A	✓	✓	✓			
B	✓		✓	✓		
C	✓	✓				✓
D		✓	✓		✓	
E				✓	✓	✓

297. A 38-year-old woman presents to the gynaecology clinic with a 6-month history of amenorrhoea and hot flushes. A pregnancy test is negative. Her serum follicle-stimulating hormone (FSH) is measured and found to be 45 IU/l.

    What further result would confirm a diagnosis of premature ovarian insufficiency (POI)?

    A. Anti-Müllerian hormone (AMH) in 2 weeks' time <1.1 pmol/l
    B. Further FSH in 2 weeks' time >50 IU/l
    C. Further FSH in 4 weeks' time >25 IU/l
    D. Immediate AMH <1.1 pmol/l
    E. Immediate luteinising hormone (LH) level >50 IU/l

298. Ulipristal acetate has previously been used for the management of uterine fibroids. What proportion of women using this treatment will develop progesterone receptor modulator-associated endometrial changes (PAEC)?

A. 10%
B. 25%
C. 40%
D. 60%
E. 90%

299. Where in the vagina is a transverse vaginal septum most commonly found?

A. Equal distribution throughout the vagina
B. Introitus
C. Lower vagina
D. Mid-vagina
E. Upper vagina

300. Which hormone is implicated in the development of endometrial polyps in obese postmenopausal women?

A. Androstenedione
B. Oestradiol
C. Oestriol
D. Oestrone
E. Testosterone

301. What are the five ultrasound parameters used to classify ovarian cysts in the risk of malignancy index (RMI)?

	Ascites	Bilateral masses	Metastases	Mixed hyper- and hypoechoic areas	Multilocular	Positive colour Doppler flow	Solid areas
A	✓	✓	✓	✓	✓		
B	✓		✓		✓	✓	✓
C		✓		✓	✓	✓	✓
D	✓	✓		✓		✓	✓
E	✓	✓	✓		✓		✓

302. A 50-year-old woman is referred to the gynaecology clinic with symptoms of abdominal bloating, loss of appetite and lower abdominal discomfort. Her serum CA125 had been measured at the GP practice and was found to be 40 IU/l. An urgent ultrasound scan is arranged, but this is reported as normal with no evidence of uterine or ovarian pathology. The patient's symptoms continue.
What is the most appropriate management?

A. Arrange urgent CT scan of pelvis
B. Arrange urgent MRI scan of pelvis
C. Assess for other clinical causes of her symptoms
D. Refer to the gynaecology multidisciplinary team meeting in view of her raised CA125
E. Repeat CA125 in 3 months' time

303. What proportion of women who have treatment with gonadotropin-releasing hormone (GnRH) analogues for the symptoms of premenstrual syndrome (PMS) will report an improvement in symptoms?

A. 5–12%
B. 22–26%
C. 31–38%
D. 45–52%
E. 60–75%

304. What is the most common benign tumour in females?

A. Breast fibroadenoma
B. Lipoma
C. Renal adenoma
D. Thyroid adenoma
E. Uterine leiomyoma

305. Which pharmacological treatment is most commonly used as a first-line therapy in the treatment of endometriosis in women with chronic pelvic pain?

A. Aromatase inhibitors
B. Combined oral contraceptive pill (COCP)
C. GnRH analogue
D. LNG-IUS
E. Oral progestogens

306. A 63-year-old woman with no significant past medical history presents with vaginal soreness, dyspareunia and dysuria, and is found to have atrophic vaginitis. She is commenced on topical vaginal oestriol cream and reports a marked improvement in her symptoms.

What advice should be given regarding the use of systemic progestogen for endometrial protection?

A. Depot medroxyprogesterone acetate every 12 weeks indefinitely
B. Insertion of LNG-IUS for duration of treatment
C. No progestogen required
D. Oral progestogen for 14 days per month
E. Transdermal progestogen for 14 days per month

307. What proportion of postmenopausal women with bleeding have co-existing cervical and endometrial polyps?

A. 4–7%
B. 14–17%
C. 24–27%
D. 34–37%
E. 44–47%

308. A woman returns to the clinic for a review following an endometrial ablation procedure and concomitant sterilisation. She is dissatisfied due to ongoing symptoms.

What are the main symptoms associated with postablation tubal sterilisation syndrome (PATSS)?

	Constant unilateral pelvic pain	Cyclical pelvic pain	Deep dyspareunia	Premature menopause	Vaginal spotting
A	✓		✓		
B		✓		✓	
C			✓		✓
D		✓			✓
E	✓			✓	

309. During an endometrial ablation procedure, what depth of myometrium needs to be destroyed to prevent endometrial regeneration from basal glands?

A. 1 mm
B. 2 mm
C. 3 mm
D. 4 mm
E. 5 mm

310. What is the most common congenital abnormality of fusion in the female genital tract?

    A. Bicornuate uterus
    B. Mayer–Rokitansky–Küster–Hauser (MRKH) syndrome
    C. Transverse vaginal septum
    D. Uterine septum
    E. Uterus didelphys

311. A 48-year-old woman presents with irregular heavy menstrual bleeding, and an endometrial biopsy confirms endometrial hyperplasia without atypia. The woman has a normal BMI and the only significant past medical history is a laparoscopic sterilisation at the age of 35. An LNG-IUS is inserted for 6 months, after which point it is removed. An endometrial biopsy at that time is normal, and a subsequent biopsy 6 months later is also normal. The woman continues to have ongoing bleeding.

    What is the appropriate management?

    A. Offer endometrial ablation
    B. Offer hysterectomy
    C. Reassure and discharge
    D. Re-insert the LNG-IUS and reassess after 1 year
    E. Repeat the endometrial biopsy after 1 year

312. What is the primary aim of medical interventions in the management of heavy menstrual bleeding?

    A. To improve haemoglobin levels
    B. To improve serum ferritin levels
    C. To improve the woman's quality of life
    D. To reduce blood loss as assessed by a menstrual calendar
    E. To reduce blood loss as assessed by pictorial charts

313. The most common cause of postmenopausal bleeding is atrophic vaginitis/endometritis.

    What is the second most common cause?

    A. Cervical polyp
    B. Endometrial carcinoma
    C. Endometrial hyperplasia
    D. Endometrial polyp
    E. Exogenous oestrogens

314. A 55-year-old woman presents with postmenopausal bleeding. A pipelle endometrial biopsy is performed, and she is found to have endometrial hyperplasia without atypia. It is explained to her that she will need to have treatment for 6 months followed by a repeat biopsy.

    Which treatment is most likely to result in a histologically normal endometrium after 6 months?

    A. Conservative management
    B. Continuous oral medroxyprogesterone acetate (MPA)
    C. Cyclical oral MPA
    D. GnRH analogues
    E. Insertion of an LNG-IUS

315. What proportion of circulating testosterone in the female is produced in the ovary?

    A. 5%
    B. 10%
    C. 15%
    D. 20%
    E. 25%

EMQs

Options for questions 316–318

A	Androgen insensitivity syndrome
B	Congenital adrenal hyperplasia
C	Imperforate hymen
D	Kallmann syndrome
E	Mayer–Rokitansky–Küster–Hauser (MRKH) syndrome
F	Polycystic ovarian syndrome (PCOS)
G	Swyer syndrome
H	Transverse vaginal septum
I	Triple X syndrome (47,XXX)
J	Turner syndrome
K	Vaginal atresia

For each of the following clinical descriptions, what is the most likely diagnosis from the option list above? Each option may be used once, more than once or not at all.

316. A 16-year-old girl presents with primary amenorrhoea. She has normal secondary sexual development. Clinical examination reveals a short, blind-ending vagina. Her karyotype is 46,XX.

317. A 15-year-old girl presents with amenorrhoea and abdominal pain. Clinical examination reveals a pelvic mass and vaginal inspection demonstrates a pink bulging membrane.

318. A 16-year-old girl presents with amenorrhoea and delayed puberty. Phenotypically, she is female and the uterus is present. Her serum FSH level is elevated. Her karyotype is 46,XY.

Options for questions 319–321

A	Chronic vulvovaginal candidiasis
B	Eczema
C	Idiopathic
D	Lichen planus
E	Lichen sclerosus
F	Lichen simplex
G	Paget's disease
H	Psoriasis
I	Recurrent herpes infection
J	Systemic lupus erythematosus
K	Vestibulodynia
L	Vulval intraepithelial neoplasia (VIN)
M	Vulvodynia

For each of the following clinical descriptions, what is the most likely diagnosis from the option list above? Each option may be used once, more than once or not at all.

319. A 58-year-old woman presents with dyspareunia, vulval itching and soreness. A biopsy is taken from atrophic areas on the vulva. The histology report states: 'There is epidermal atrophy, hyperkeratosis with subepidermal hyalinisation of collagen and lichenoid infiltrate.'

320. A 23-year-old woman with schizophrenia presents with vaginal itch and soreness. On examination, there are marked excoriations and lichenification. Most of her pubic hair is absent.

321. A 40-year-old woman presents with vaginal soreness, discharge and dyspareunia. On examination, the mucosal surfaces of the vagina are eroded. At the edges of the erosions, the epithelium is mauve/grey, and Wickham's striae are noted.

Options for questions 322–324

A	Combined oral contraceptive pill (COCP)
B	Daily progestogen on days 5–25 of cycle
C	Daily progestogen in the luteal phase
D	Danazol
E	Etamsylate
F	GnRH agonist
G	Hysteroscopic myomectomy
H	Levonorgestrel-releasing intrauterine system (LNG-IUS)
I	Mefenamic acid
J	No treatment required
K	Open myomectomy
L	Second-generation endometrial ablation
M	Subtotal hysterectomy
N	Total abdominal hysterectomy
O	Tranexamic acid
P	Transcervical resection of endometrium

For each of the following clinical scenarios, what would be the most appropriate treatment option from the list above? Each option may be used once, more than once or not at all.

322. A 38-year-old woman with heavy menstrual bleeding is seen in the gynaecology clinic. Her medical history is unremarkable other than mild renal impairment. The woman is keen to avoid hormonal treatments.

323. A 35-year-old woman attends the gynaecology clinic with heavy menstrual bleeding and dysmenorrhoea. Her history is otherwise unremarkable, but a pelvic examination demonstrates an enlarged uterus with possible fibroids. A pelvic ultrasound scan is arranged, but the woman is desperate to start treatment immediately.

324. A 37-year-old woman with a BMI of 38 kg/m^2 returns to the clinic for a review. She is para 2+0 and her family is complete. Her husband has had a vasectomy. Six months earlier, she had an LNG-IUS inserted for heavy menstrual bleeding, but this has recently been removed by the GP due to persistent vaginal bleeding. Prior to this she had already tried tranexamic acid and mefenamic acid without effect. A previous pelvic examination suggested an enlarged uterus (equivalent to 9 weeks of gestation), and a subsequent ultrasound scan demonstrated multiple small (<2 cm) intramural fibroids.

Options for questions 325–327

A	Cervical smear
B	Coagulation tests
C	CT scan
D	Full blood count (FBC)
E	Hysteroscopy
F	MRI scan
G	No investigation required
H	Pelvic ultrasound scan
I	Pipelle endometrial biopsy
J	Serum ferritin
K	Serum follicle-stimulating hormone (FSH)
L	Serum oestradiol
M	Three-dimensional ultrasound scan
N	Thyroid function tests

For each of the following clinical scenarios, what would be the next most appropriate investigation from the options above? Each option may be used once, more than once or not at all.

325. A 39-year-old woman with a BMI of 40 kg/m^2 attends the gynaecology clinic with heavy menstrual bleeding. Her medical history is unremarkable and an FBC taken by the referring GP was normal. Examination is difficult due to the woman's size.

326. A 27-year-old woman attends the GP surgery with heavy menstrual bleeding that is affecting her quality of life. Her history and examination are unremarkable.

327. A 44-year-old woman presents to the clinic with heavy menstrual bleeding and intermittent but ongoing intermenstrual bleeding. Her smear history is normal. She describes recurrent episodes of vaginal thrush but has no other medical problems.

Options for questions 328–330

A	Cognitive behavioural therapy (CBT)
B	Continuous combined hormone replacement therapy (HRT)
C	Cyclical norethisterone
D	Danazol
E	Drospirenone-containing combined oral contraceptive pill (COCP)
F	Evening primrose oil
G	GnRH analogue
H	LNG-IUS
I	Micronised progesterone
J	Norethisterone
K	Norethisterone-containing COCP
L	Selective serotonin reuptake inhibitors (SSRIs)
M	Spironolactone
N	Tibolone
O	Transdermal oestradiol
P	Vitamin B6

For each of the following clinical scenarios, what would be the most appropriate treatment option from the list above? Each option may be used once, more than once or not at all.

328. A 28-year-old woman presents to clinic with symptoms suggestive of premenstrual syndrome (PMS). She subsequently returns for a review appointment after 2 months of completing a symptom diary, but the completed diary does not give a clear diagnosis. What treatment should be considered for 3 months to facilitate a definitive diagnosis?

329. An otherwise healthy 30-year-old woman with a BMI of 24 kg/m² has completed a symptom diary that is strongly suggestive of a diagnosis of PMS. What would be considered the first-line pharmaceutical treatment option?

330. A 42-year-old woman with severe PMS opts to have a laparoscopic bilateral oophorectomy following failed medical management. She decided to retain her uterus and has commenced transdermal oestrogen therapy. What would be considered the optimal first-line therapy for endometrial protection?

Options for questions 331 and 332

A	Atrophic vaginitis
B	Bacterial vaginosis
C	Candidiasis
D	Cervical ectropion
E	Cervical polyp
F	*Chlamydia* infection
G	Endometrial polyp
H	Fallopian tube carcinoma
I	Gonorrhoea
J	Physiological discharge
K	Trichomoniasis
L	Urethral caruncle
M	Vaginal carcinoma

For each of the following clinical scenarios, what is the most likely cause for the vaginal discharge described from the options above? Each option may be used once, more than once or not at all.

331. A 26-year-old woman presents with a complaint of recurrent vaginal discharge. A gynaecological examination is unremarkable. High vaginal and endocervical swabs are taken for microbiological testing but results are awaited.

332. A 35-year-old woman presents to the GP practice with an offensive vaginal discharge. The discharge is associated with dysuria and vulval itching.

Options for questions 333–335

A	Amitriptyline
B	Codeine
C	Co-dydramol
D	Combined oral contraceptive pill (COCP)
E	Danazol
F	Fluoxetine
G	Gabapentin
H	Glycerin suppositories
I	GnRH analogue
J	Ibuprofen
K	Lactulose
L	Mebeverine
M	No treatment required
N	Paracetamol
O	Paroxetine
P	Peppermint water
Q	Senna
R	Sertraline

For each of the following clinical scenarios, what would be the most appropriate first-line pharmacological treatment from the options above? Each option may be used once, more than once or not at all.

333. A 22-year-old woman presents with an 8-month history of significant intermittent abdominal pain. Her menstrual cycle is irregular. She has noted an increase in frequency in passing stools. The pain seems to improve after defecation.

334. A 20-year-old woman presents with a 2-year history of chronic pelvic pain. The pain is present on most days but is worse around the time of menstruation. She has noted that her stools are more firm than previously. She does not have urinary frequency.

335. A 30-year-old woman with a BMI of 25 kg/m^2 presents to the clinic with cyclical chronic pelvic pain. An ultrasound scan is normal. At her insistence, a diagnostic laparoscopy is performed, which shows no obvious pathology. She has completed symptoms charts, which show a distinct cyclical pattern to her symptoms.

Options for questions 336–338

A	Combined oral contraceptive pill (COCP)
B	GnRH analogue
C	Laparoscopic bilateral oophorectomy
D	Laparoscopic ovarian cystectomy
E	Laparoscopic unilateral oophorectomy
F	Laparoscopy and ovarian cyst aspiration
G	Laparotomy and bilateral oophorectomy
H	Laparotomy and ovarian cystectomy
I	Laparotomy, bilateral oophorectomy and omental biopsy
J	No treatment required
K	Total abdominal hysterectomy and bilateral salpingo-oophorectomy
L	Ultrasound-guided ovarian cyst aspiration

For each of the following clinical scenarios, what would be the most appropriate management from the options listed? Each option may be used once, more than once or not at all.

336. A 45-year-old woman has an incidental finding of an ovarian cyst during an MRI scan for lower back pain. The following month, an ultrasound scan is arranged by the GP, which reports a simple 4 cm cyst in the left ovary. The remainder of the pelvic ultrasound scan is normal.

337. A 26-year-old woman with a BMI of 30 kg/m^2 who has never been pregnant presents with an ache in the right side of the pelvis. A transvaginal ultrasound scan reports a 10 cm complex mass in the right adnexa with appearances compatible with a dermoid cyst. Tumour markers are all normal.

338. A 49-year-old woman with a BMI of 25 kg/m^2 presents with left-sided abdominal pain and bloating. She is having a regular menstrual cycle. A detailed history reveals that she has urinary frequency. A transvaginal ultrasound scan reports a simple 8 cm cyst in the left ovary. Tumour markers are normal.

Options for questions 339 and 340

A	Adrenocortical adenocarcinoma
B	Adrenocortical adenoma
C	Congenital adrenal hyperplasia
D	Cushing's disease
E	Cushing's syndrome
F	Exogenous androgens
G	Gestational hyperandrogenism
H	Idiopathic
I	Ovarian hyperthecosis
J	Polycystic ovarian syndrome (PCOS)
K	Sertoli–Leydig cell tumour

For each of the following clinical scenarios, what is the most likely cause of hyper-androgenism from the options listed? Each option may be used once, more than once or not at all.

339. A 25-year-old woman presents with excessive facial hair and acne vulgaris.

340. A 65-year-old woman presents with persistent coarse facial hair. Blood tests reveal she has hyperandrogenaemia.

Answers
SBAs

291. Answer **C** Endometrial biopsy at 6 and 12 months and discharge if normal

Explanation
Endometrial surveillance should be arranged at a minimum of 6-monthly intervals, although review schedules should be individualised and responsive to changes in a woman's clinical condition. At least two consecutive 6-monthly negative biopsies should be obtained prior to discharge. In women at higher risk of relapse, such as women with a BMI of $\geq$35 kg/m^2 or those treated with oral progestogens, 6-monthly endometrial biopsies are recommended. Once two consecutive negative endometrial biopsies have been obtained, then long-term follow-up should be considered with annual endometrial biopsies.

Reference

RCOG. Management of endometrial hyperplasia. *RCOG GTG No. 67.* February 2016.

292. Answer **A** Arrange a follow-up ultrasound scan in 4 months

Explanation
Simple, unilateral, unilocular ovarian cysts of <5 cm in diameter have a low risk of malignancy. It is recommended that, in the presence of normal serum CA125 levels, they be managed conservatively. Numerous studies have looked at the risk of malignancy in ovarian cysts, comparing ultrasound morphology with either histology at subsequent surgery or by close follow-up of those women managed conservatively. The risk of malignancy in these studies of cysts that are <5 cm, unilateral, unilocular and echo-free with no solid parts or papillary formations is <1%. In addition, >50% of these cysts will resolve spontaneously within 3 months. Thus, it is reasonable to manage these cysts conservatively, with a follow-up ultrasound scan for cysts of 2–5 cm, a reasonable interval being 4 months. This, of course, depends on the views and symptoms of the woman and on the gynaecologist's clinical assessment.

Reference

RCOG. Ovarian cysts in postmenopausal women. *RCOG GTG No. 34.* July 2016.

293. Answer **C** Insertion of an LNG-IUS

Explanation
Consider an LNG-IUS as the first treatment for heavy menstrual bleeding in women with suspected or diagnosed adenomyosis.

Reference

NICE. Heavy menstrual bleeding: assessment and management. *NICE Guideline (NG88).* March 2018.

294. Answer **B** Six cycles

Explanation
Women offered an LNG-IUS should be advised of anticipated changes in the bleeding pattern, particularly in the first few cycles and possibly lasting >6 months. They should therefore be advised to persevere for at least six cycles to see the benefits of the treatment.

Reference
NICE. Heavy menstrual bleeding: assessment and management. *NICE Guideline (NG88)*. March 2018.

295. Answer **B** Erosive

Explanation
The anogenital lesions of lichen planus may be divided into three main groups according to their clinical presentation:

- Classical
- Hypertrophic
- Erosive.

Erosive is the most common subtype to cause vulval symptoms.

Reference
Edwards SK, Bates CM, Lewis F, Sethi G, Grover D. 2014 UK national guideline on the management of vulval conditions. *International Journal of STD & AIDS* 2015;26:611–24.

296. Answer **B** Chronic pelvic pain, deep dyspareunia and dysmenorrhoea

Explanation
Dysmenorrhoea was the chief complaint, reported by 62% of women with mainly peritoneal endometriosis in a Brazilian study by Bellelis *et al.* (2010; cited in the reference article). In the same study, the prevalence of chronic pelvic pain was 57%, deep dyspareunia 55%, cyclic intestinal complaints 48%, infertility 40% and incapacitating dysmenorrhoea 28%.

Reference
ESHRE. Management of women with endometriosis. *ESHRE Guideline*. September 2013.

297. Answer **C** Further FSH in 4 weeks' time >25 IU/l

Explanation
Although proper diagnostic accuracy in POI is lacking, the guideline development group recommends the following two diagnostic criteria:

- Oligo/amenorrhoea for at least 4 months, and
- An elevated FSH level >25 IU/l on two occasions >4 weeks apart.

Reference
ESHRE. Management of women with premature ovarian insufficiency. *ESHRE Guideline*. December 2015.

298. **Answer** **D** 60%

Explanation
Ulipristal acetate use has been found to be associated with benign endometrial changes termed PAEC. These changes were noted in up to two-thirds of women during treatment and resolved within 6 months of discontinuation of treatment.

Reference

Younas K, Hadoura E, Majoko F, Bunkheila A. A review of evidence-based management of uterine fibroids. *The Obstetrician & Gynaecologist* 2016;18:33–42.

299. **Answer** **E** Upper vagina

Explanation
The incidence of this is unclear but is probably not greater than 1 in 30,000 to 1 in 50,000. The septae may occur anywhere along the length of the vagina, although they are classified as upper, mid- and lower, with the upper septae accounting for 46%, the mid-vagina 30–40% and the lower vagina 15–20%.

Reference

Edmonds DK, Rose GL. Outflow tract disorders of the female genital tract. *The Obstetrician & Gynaecologist* 2013;15:11–17.

300. **Answer** **D** Oestrone

Explanation
In obese women, it is the increased circulating level of oestrone that is likely to be the cause of polyp development and growth.

Reference

Otify M, Fuller J, Ross J, Shaikh H, Johns J. Endometrial pathology in the postmenopausal woman – an evidence based approach to management. *The Obstetrician & Gynaecologist* 2015;17:29–38.

301. **Answer** **E**

Explanation
RMI is calculated as: RMI = $U \times M \times$ CA125, where $U = 0$ (for an ultrasound score of 0), $U = 1$ (for an ultrasound score of 1) or $U = 3$ (for ultrasound score of 2–5); $M = 3$ for all postmenopausal women dealt with by this guideline; and CA125 is the serum CA125 measurement in IU/ml.

Ultrasound scans score 1 point for each of the following characteristics:

- Multilocular cyst
- Evidence of solid areas
- Evidence of metastases
- Presence of ascites
- Bilateral lesions.

Reference

RCOG. Ovarian cysts in postmenopausal women. *RCOG GTG No. 34*. July 2016.

302.   Answer   C   Assess for other clinical causes of her symptoms

Explanation
A woman with normal serum CA125 level (<35 IU/ml), or with CA125 of
≥35 IU/ml but a normal ultrasound should be assessed carefully for other clinical
causes of her symptoms and investigated if appropriate. If no other clinical cause
is apparent, she should be advised to return to her GP if her symptoms become
more frequent and/or persistent.

Reference

NICE. Ovarian cancer: recognition and initial management. *NICE Clinical Guideline
(CG122)*. April 2011.

303.   Answer   E   60–75%

Explanation
Several randomised controlled trials have demonstrated improvement of PMS
symptoms, with a response rate to GnRH analogue treatment of between 60% and
75%.

Reference

Walsh S, Ismaili E, Naheed B, O'Brien S. Diagnosis, pathophysiology and management of
premenstrual syndrome. *The Obstetrician & Gynaecologist* 2015;17:99–104.

304.   Answer   E   Uterine leiomyoma

Explanation
Uterine fibroids (leiomyomata) are the most type of common benign tumour in
women, with a lifetime prevalence of around 30%.

Reference

Younas K, Hadoura E, Majoko F, Bunkheila A. A review of evidence-based management of
uterine fibroids. *The Obstetrician & Gynaecologist* 2016;18:33–42.

305.   Answer   B   Combined oral contraceptive pill (COCP)

Explanation
Commonly used hormonal therapies include the combined contraceptive pill,
GnRH analogues, progestogens (via different routes, including an LNG-IUS and
injectable progestogens) and, less commonly, aromatase inhibitors. Combined
oral contraceptives have been shown to produce similar results to GnRH
analogues in the management of chronic pelvic pain in these women, and thus,
with their lower adverse effect profile, are more frequently used as a first-line
therapy.

Reference

Issa B, Ormesher L, Whorwell PJ, Shah M, Hamdy S. Endometriosis and irritable bowel
syndrome: a dilemma for the gynaecologist and gastroenterologist. *The Obstetrician &
Gynaecologist* 2016;18:9–16.

306. Answer **C** No progestogen required

   Explanation
   Systemic absorption is insignificant with low-dose topical oestrogen. Additional systemic progestogen is not required.

   ### Reference
   Bakour SH, Williamson J. Latest evidence on using hormone replacement therapy in the menopause. *The Obstetrician & Gynaecologist* 2015;17:20–8.

307. Answer **C** 24–27%

   Explanation
   Co-existing cervical and endometrial polyps will be present in 24–27% of women at presentation.

   ### Reference
   Otify M, Fuller J, Ross J, Shaikh H, Johns J. Endometrial pathology in the postmenopausal woman – an evidence based approach to management. *The Obstetrician & Gynaecologist* 2015;17:29–38.

308. Answer **D** Cyclical pelvic pain, and vaginal spotting

   Explanation
   PATSS is a recognised complication known to occur in cases where sterilisation is combined with ablation. The main symptoms are cyclical unilateral/bilateral pelvic pain with vaginal spotting. The mechanism of pain is thought to be retrograde menstruation into the obstructed fallopian tube resulting in distension of the fallopian tubes. The incidence varies from 6% to 8%.

   ### Reference
   Saraswat L, Cooper K. Surgical management of heavy menstrual bleeding: part 1. *The Obstetrician & Gynaecologist* 2017;19:37–45.

309. Answer **E** 5 mm

   Explanation
   The endometrium is known for its remarkable ability to regenerate. Full-thickness destruction of the endometrium along with superficial myometrium to 5 mm, which contains basal endometrial glands, is required to stop menstrual flow. Regeneration from these basal glands is often a reason for treatment failure.

   ### Reference
   Saraswat L, Cooper K. Surgical management of heavy menstrual bleeding: part 1. *The Obstetrician & Gynaecologist* 2017;19:37–45.

310. Answer **D** Uterine septum

   Explanation
   The incidence of congenital anomalies of the genital tract is difficult to determine, as many women with anomalies are not diagnosed if they are not symptomatic.

These abnormalities are primarily abnormalities of uterine fusion with septate uteri constituting 90% of cases, bicornuate uteri 5%, and the didelphic uterus 5%, when the abnormality is detected.

Reference

Edmonds DK, Rose GL. Outflow tract disorders of the female genital tract. *The Obstetrician & Gynaecologist* 2013;15:11–7.

311. Answer   **B**   Offer hysterectomy

Explanation
Hysterectomy is indicated in women not wanting to preserve their fertility when there is any one of the following:

- Progression to atypical hyperplasia occurs during follow-up
- There is no histological regression of hyperplasia, despite 12 months of treatment
- There is relapse of endometrial hyperplasia after completing progestogen treatment
- There is persistence of bleeding symptoms
- The woman declines to undergo endometrial surveillance or comply with medical treatment.

Reference

RCOG. Management of endometrial hyperplasia. *RCOG GTG No. 67.* February 2016.

312. Answer   **C**   To improve the woman's quality of life

Explanation
It should be recognised that heavy menstrual bleeding has a major impact on a woman's quality of life, and any intervention should aim to improve this rather than focusing on blood loss.

Reference

NICE. Heavy menstrual bleeding: assessment and management. *NICE Guideline (NG88).* March 2018.

313. Answer   **E**   Exogenous oestrogens

Pathological findings in women with postmenopausal bleeding are:

Endometrial/cervical polyps	2–12%
Endometrial hyperplasia	5–10%
Endometrial carcinoma	10%
Exogenous oestrogens	15–25%
Atrophic vaginitis/endometritis	60–80%

Reference

Otify M, Fuller J, Ross J, Shaikh H, Johns J. Endometrial pathology in the postmenopausal woman – an evidence based approach to management. *The Obstetrician & Gynaecologist* 2015;17:29–38.

314. Answer   E   Insertion of an LNG-IUS

Explanation
A recent multicentre randomised trial compared the treatment of endometrial hyperplasia with LNG-IUS, oral MPA 10 mg administered for 10 days per cycle or continuous oral MPA 10 mg daily, for 6 months. The LNG-IUS-treated group achieved a 100% histologically normal endometrium after 6 months of therapy, while this value was 96% and 69% for women in the continuous oral group and cyclical progestogen group, respectively.

Reference

Otify M, Fuller J, Ross J, Shaikh H, Johns J. Endometrial pathology in the postmenopausal woman – an evidence based approach to management. *The Obstetrician & Gynaecologist* 2015;17:29–38.

315. Answer   E   25%

Explanation
The ovary also produces and releases androgens, including 20% of dehydroepiandrosterone, 50% of androstenedione and 25% of circulating testosterone.

Reference

Meek CL, Bravis V, Don A, Kaplan F. Polycystic ovary syndrome and the differential diagnosis of hyperandrogenism. *The Obstetrician & Gynaecologist* 2013;15:171–6.

EMQs

316. Answer   E   Mayer–Rokitansky–Küster–Hauser (MRKH) syndrome

Explanation
MRKH syndrome (Müllerian agenesis) is a malformation complex characterised by congenital absence of the upper two-thirds of the vagina and an absent or rudimentary uterus in women who have normal development of secondary sexual characteristics and a 46,XX karyotype.

Reference

Valappil S, Chetan U, Wood N, Garden A. Mayer–Rokitansky–Küster–Hauser syndrome: diagnosis and management. *The Obstetrician & Gynaecologist* 2012;14:93–8.

317. Answer   H   Transverse vaginal septum

Explanation
In an imperforate hymen, inspection of the vulva reveals a membrane that is blue in appearance with the darkened blood transilluminating through the thin membrane. A differential diagnosis of a transverse vaginal septum must always be considered, but the appearances here are totally different, with the septum being pink, although bulging, because the septum is so much thicker.

Reference

Edmonds DK, Rose GL. Outflow tract disorders of the female genital tract. *The Obstetrician & Gynaecologist* 2013;15:11–7.

318. Answer   **G**   Swyer syndrome

Explanation
Swyer syndrome is a form of gonadal dysgenesis where the karyotype is 46,XY. The streak gonads do not make androgens so the person is phenotypically female. As there is no hormone feedback to the hypothalamus/pituitary, FSH is elevated. The streak gonads do not make Müllerian inhibitory factor so the uterus is present (it would be absent in androgen insensitivity syndrome).

Reference
Garden A, Hernon M, Topping J (eds*.*). *Paediatric and Adolescent Gynaecology for the MRCOG and Beyond*, 2nd edn. London: RCOG Press, 2012, p. 57.

319. Answer   **E**   Lichen sclerosus

Explanation
The histology of a vulval biopsy for vulval lichen sclerosus is a thinned epidermis with subepidermal hyalinisation and deeper inflammatory infiltrate. Although the diagnosis of lichen sclerosus is usually made on clinical findings, this is a textbook definition of histopathological findings from a vulval biopsy.

320. Answer   **F**   Lichen simplex

Explanation
Lichen simplex is categorised into four main categories, of which psychiatric disorders is one. There may be a chronic itch–scratch cycle, which results in lichenification and often loss of pubic hair.

321. Answer   **D**   Lichen planus

Explanation
The anogenital lesions of lichen planus may be divided into three main groups according to their clinical presentation: classical, hypertrophic and erosive.
    Erosive is the most common subtype to cause vulval symptoms. The mucosal surfaces are eroded, and at the edges of the erosions, the epithelium is mauve and a pale network (Wickham's striae) is sometimes seen.

Reference
Edwards SK, Bates CM, Lewis F, Sethi G, Grover D. 2014 UK national guideline on the management of vulval conditions. *International Journal of STD & AIDS* 2015;26:611–24.

322. Answer   **O**   Tranexamic acid

Explanation
If a woman with heavy menstrual bleeding declines an LNG-IUS or it is not suitable, consider the following pharmacological treatments:
Non-hormonal:

- Tranexamic acid
- Non-steroidal anti-inflammatory drugs (NSAIDs).

Hormonal:

- Combined hormonal contraception
- Cyclical oral progestogens.

Her history and examination suggest that pharmaceutical options are appropriate; however, most treatment options are hormonal. NSAIDs should be avoided with a history of renal impairment.

323. Answer   **I**   Mefenamic acid

Explanation
If pharmaceutical treatment is required while investigations and definitive treatment are being organised, either tranexamic acid or NSAIDs (such as mefenamic acid) should be used. When heavy menstrual bleeding co-exists with dysmenorrhoea, NSAIDs may be more effective than tranexamic acid.

324. Answer   **L**   Second-generation endometrial ablation

Explanation
If treatment for heavy menstrual bleeding is unsuccessful, the woman declines pharmacological treatment or symptoms are severe, consider referral to specialist care for investigations to diagnose the cause of the heavy bleeding, if needed taking into account any investigations the woman has already had and alternative treatment choices, including pharmacological options not already tried, and surgical options, such as second-generation endometrial ablation or a hysterectomy.

In view of the woman's raised BMI, it would be preferable to try endometrial ablation in the first instance, rather than a hysterectomy.

Reference

NICE. Heavy menstrual bleeding: assessment and management. *NICE Guideline (NG88).* March 2018.

325. Answer   **H**   Pelvic ultrasound scan

Explanation
Offer a pelvic ultrasound to women with heavy menstrual bleeding if any of the following apply:

- Their uterus is palpable abdominally
- Their history or examination suggests a pelvic mass
- Examination is inconclusive or difficult, for example in women who are obese.

326. Answer   **D**   Full blood count (FBC)

An FBC should be carried out on all women with heavy menstrual bleeding. This should be done in parallel with any heavy menstrual bleeding treatment offered.

327. Answer   **E**   Hysteroscopy

Offer an outpatient hysteroscopy to women with heavy menstrual bleeding if their history suggests submucosal fibroids, polyps or endometrial pathology because:

- They have symptoms such as persistent intermenstrual bleeding or
- They have risk factors for endometrial pathology.

Reference

NICE. Heavy menstrual bleeding: assessment and management. *NICE Guideline (NG88)*. March 2018.

328. Answer   **G**   GnRH analogue

Explanation
GnRH analogues may be used for 3 months for a definitive diagnosis if the completed symptom diary alone is inconclusive.

329. Answer   **E**   Drospirenone-containing combined oral contraceptive pill (COCP)

Explanation
When treating women with PMS, the drospirenone-containing COCP may represent effective treatment and should be considered as a first-line pharmaceutical intervention.

330. Answer   **I**   Micronised progesterone

Explanation
Micronised progesterone is theoretically less likely to reintroduce PMS-like symptoms and should therefore be considered as a first-line treatment for progestogenic opposition rather than progestogens.

Reference

RCOG. Management of premenstrual syndrome. *RCOG GTG No. 48*. December 2016.

331. Answer   **B**   Bacterial vaginosis

Bacterial vaginosis is the commonest cause of abnormal vaginal discharge.

332. Answer   **K**   Trichomoniasis

Explanation
The symptoms are suggestive of trichomoniasis. *Chlamydia* infection and gonorrhoea are less likely due to the patient's age and are not usually associated with vaginal itching.

Reference

Lazaro N. Sexually transmitted infections in primary care. *RCGP/BASHH*. 2013.

333.   Answer   **L**   Mebeverine

Explanation
This woman has irritable bowel syndrome according to the Rome III criteria.
A systematic review concluded that smooth muscle relaxants such as mebeverine hydrochloride are beneficial in the treatment of irritable bowel syndrome where abdominal pain is a prominent feature. The efficacy of bulking agents has not been established, but they are commonly used.

334.   Answer   **D**   Combined oral contraceptive pill (COCP)

Explanation
This woman's symptoms are suggestive of endometriosis. She does not meet the criteria for irritable bowel syndrome. A therapeutic trial of hormonal treatment should be offered. The COCP is the most appropriate option. GnRH agonists will render her hypo-oestrogenic, which is not appropriate at the age of 20. Danazol is associated with masculinising side effects.

335.   Answer   **D**   Combined oral contraceptive pill (COCP)

Explanation
Ovarian suppression can be an effective treatment for cyclical pain associated with endometriosis. The effect can be achieved with the COCP, progestogens, danazol or GnRH analogues, all of which are equally effective but have differing adverse effect profiles.
Non-endometriosis-related cyclical pain also appears to be well controlled by these treatments.
This woman is young with a normal BMI. The COCP will be associated with the fewest side effects for her.

Reference
RCOG. The initial management of chronic pelvic pain. *RCOG GTG No. 41*. May 2012.

336.   Answer   **J**   No treatment required

Explanation
Women with small (<50 mm diameter) simple ovarian cysts generally do not require follow-up as these cysts are very likely to be physiological and almost always resolve within three menstrual cycles.

337.   Answer   **H**   Laparotomy and ovarian cystectomy

Explanation
In the presence of large masses with solid components (e.g. large dermoid cysts), laparotomy may be appropriate. This is a young woman who has not been pregnant, so it would be preferable to conserve any normal ovarian tissue if possible.

338. Answer   **E**   Laparoscopic unilateral oophorectomy

Explanation
Cysts >70 mm in diameter should be considered for either further imaging (MRI) or surgical intervention due to difficulties in examining the entire cyst adequately at the time of ultrasound.

The laparoscopic approach for elective surgical management of ovarian masses presumed to be benign is associated with lower postoperative morbidity and shorter recovery time, and is preferred to laparotomy in suitable patients.

This woman is symptomatic, and her urinary frequency may be related to pressure effects of the cyst. Surgery is therefore preferable to further imaging. An oophorectomy will be a simpler operation with less chance of spillage of the cyst contents.

An argument could be made for a bilateral oophorectomy as the women is close to menopausal age, but if the remaining ovary is normal, there is no clear justification for removing it.

Reference

RCOG. Management of suspected ovarian masses in premenopausal women. *RCOG GTG No. 62.* December 2011.

339. Answer   **J**   Polycystic ovarian syndrome (PCOS)

Explanation
PCOS is the most common cause of hyperandrogenism in women of reproductive age.

340. Answer   **I**   Ovarian hyperthecosis

Explanation
Ovarian hyperthecosis accounts for most of the cases of hyperandrogenaemia in postmenopausal women.

Reference

Meek CL, Bravis V, Don A, Kaplan F. Polycystic ovary syndrome and the differential diagnosis of hyperandrogenism. *The Obstetrician & Gynaecologist* 2013;15:171–6.

Subfertility

SBAs

341. A woman is diagnosed with hyperthyroidism as part of fertility investigations and opts to have treatment with radioactive iodine.
   What is the minimum time she should delay conception after radioactive iodine treatment?

   A. 2 weeks
   B. 1 month
   C. 3 months
   D. 6 months
   E. 12 months

342. What is the most common cause of testicular failure?

   A. Idiopathic
   B. Klinefelter's syndrome
   C. Radiotherapy
   D. Varicocele
   E. Y chromosome microdeletions

343. One hundred couples are investigated for failure to conceive after 1 year of regular unprotected intercourse.
   What proportion of these couples will have unexplained infertility?

   A. 15%
   B. 25%
   C. 35%
   D. 45%
   E. 55%

344. What is the single most important factor in determining female reproductive outcome?

   A. Female age
   B. Ovarian antral follicle count
   C. Previous pregnancy
   D. Serum anti-Müllerian hormone (AMH)
   E. Serum follicle-stimulating hormone (FSH) in the early follicular phase

345. What is the most frequently used test of ovarian reserve?
   A. Basal FSH in the early follicular phase
   B. Clomifene citrate challenge test
   C. Ovarian antral follicle count
   D. Serum AMH
   E. Serum inhibin B

346. During the course of fertility investigations, a 34-year-old woman has an ultrasound scan that suggests the presence of adenomyosis. All other investigations are normal, and the partner's semen analysis is satisfactory. The couple have been trying to conceive for 1 year.
   What is the optimal management?
   A. Diagnostic laparoscopy to confirm the diagnosis
   B. Explain that there is no known association between adenomyosis and subfertility
   C. Hysteroscopic resection of the adenomyosis
   D. Offer in vitro fertilisation (IVF) treatment
   E. Treat with gonadotropin-releasing hormone (GnRH) analogues

347. During the course of fertility investigations, a 35-year-old woman has an ultrasound scan that shows the presence of three intramural fibroids, each measuring 2 cm in diameter.
   What is the optimal management?
   A. Conservative management
   B. GnRH analogues for 6 months
   C. Hysteroscopic myomectomy
   D. Laparoscopic myomectomy
   E. Open myomectomy

348. What is the best test of fallopian tube function?
   A. Hystero-contrast-salpingography (HyCoSy)
   B. Hysterosalpingogram (HSG)
   C. Laparoscopy and dye test
   D. Rubin's test
   E. Spontaneous intrauterine pregnancy

349. Which cell type is the end product of meiosis in the testes?
   A. Leydig cell
   B. Primary spermatocyte
   C. Secondary spermatocyte
   D. Spermatid
   E. Spermatogonium

350. What proportion of infertility is thought to be attributable to male factors?

    A. 10%
    B. 30%
    C. 50%
    D. 70%
    E. 90%

351. Which cases of ovarian hyperstimulation syndrome (OHSS) should be reported to the HFEA?

    A. All cases of OHSS
    B. Only cases of critical OHSS
    C. Only cases of moderate, severe and critical OHSS
    D. Only cases of severe and critical OHSS
    E. Only cases of severe OHSS

352. Which analgesic should be avoided in women presenting with OHSS?

    A. Codeine
    B. Ibuprofen
    C. Morphine
    D. Paracetamol
    E. Pethidine

353. Following IVF treatment in which 15 oocytes were collected, a woman attends the gynaecology emergency unit with mild lower abdominal pain and bloating. Her GP suspects the presence of OHSS. An ultrasound scan is performed. The mean ovarian diameter is 6 cm. There is no evidence of ascites.
    What type of OHSS is this?

    A. Critical OHSS
    B. Mild OHSS
    C. Moderate OHSS
    D. Severe OHSS
    E. This is not OHSS

354. What is the most appropriate management of hydrosalpinges prior to IVF treatment?

    A. Conservative management
    B. Laparoscopic salpingectomy
    C. Laparoscopic salpingostomy
    D. Laparoscopic tubal clipping
    E. Ultrasound-guided drainage

355. A woman who has had three previous IVF treatments is diagnosed with recurrent implantation failure and opts to have an endometrial scratch (endometrial injury) as part of her upcoming treatment?

    When should this be performed in relation to the IVF treatment cycle?

    A. At the onset of menstruation, immediately before the start of ovarian stimulation
    B. 7 days prior to the onset of menstruation, immediately before the start of ovarian stimulation
    C. 14 days prior to the onset of menstruation, immediately before the start of ovarian stimulation
    D. 21 days prior to the onset of menstruation, immediately before the start of ovarian stimulation
    E. 7 days after the onset of menstruation, during ovarian stimulation

EMQs

Options for questions 356–358

A	Daily follicle-stimulating hormone (FSH) injections
B	Donated embryos
C	Donor insemination
D	Intracytoplasmic sperm injection (ICSI)
E	ICSI with donated eggs
F	ICSI with donor eggs and donor sperm
G	Intrauterine insemination with donor sperm
H	Intrauterine insemination with partner sperm
I	In vitro fertilisation (IVF)
J	IVF with donor eggs and donor sperm
K	No treatment required
L	Ovulation induction and donor insemination
M	Ovulation induction and donor intrauterine insemination
N	Ovualtion induction with clomifene
O	Surgical sperm retrieval followed by ICSI
P	Surgical sperm retrieval followed by intrauterine insemination
Q	Surgical sperm retrieval followed by IVF

For each of the following clinical scenarios, what is the most appropriate treatment option from the list above? Each option may be used once, more than once or not at all.

356. A 46-year-old woman presents to the IVF clinic with her new partner. She wishes to become pregnant. Her menstrual cycle is irregular with a duration of 28–45 days, with periods lasting 1–2 days. Her serum FSH is 18.7 IU/l and her AMH level is <1.1 pmol/l. A pelvic ultrasound scan is normal.
Her partner's semen analysis results are:

Semen count analysis:	8.3×10^6/ml
Progressive motility	11%
Morphology	2%

357. A couple attend the fertility clinic. The woman has irregular periods and clinical evidence of hyperandrogenism. Her AMH level is 67 pmol/l. An HSG confirms patent fallopian tubes. The man has azoospermia. In the past, he has been investigated and a testicular biopsy showed maturation arrest.

358. A couple are referred to the fertility clinic for investigation. The woman is 32 years of age and has no significant past medical history. She has a regular 28-day cycle. The man is 34 years of age and has a history of orchidopexy as a child for a left undescended testis. He has two semen analyses, both of which are normal. The woman's results are:

Day 2 FSH	4.5 IU/l
Day 21 progesterone	35 nmol/l
Pelvic ultrasound scan	Normal
HSG	Normal cavity, bilateral patent tubes

Options for questions 359–361

A	Anastrozole
B	Bromocriptine
C	Cabergoline
D	Clomifene citrate
E	Follicle-stimulating hormone (FSH) injections
F	Human chorionic gonadotropin (hCG) injections
G	Laparoscopic ovarian drilling
H	Letrozole
I	Metformin
J	No treatment required
K	Oral cetrorelix
L	Oral progestogen for 10 days
M	Ovarian wedge resection
N	Tamoxifen
O	Weight gain
P	Weight loss

For each of the following clinical scenarios, what is the most appropriate treatment option from the list above? Each option may be used once, more than once or not at all.

359. During the course of fertility investigations, a 28-year-old woman with a BMI of 35 kg/m² is found to have polycystic ovaries on ultrasound scanning. Her menstrual cycle has a length of 35–70 days. Her partner's semen analysis is normal.

360. A 32-year-old woman and her husband present to the clinic with 1 year of subfertility. Investigations show them to have unexplained infertility. The woman requests treatment as she has read on the internet that there are drugs that can be used to 'boost fertility'.

361. A woman with a BMI of 28 kg/m² and polycystic ovarian syndrome (PCOS) has attempted ovulation induction with clomifene citrate without success. She now returns to the clinic with pelvic pain that is worse around the time of menstruation.

Options for questions 362–364

A	Serum androstenedione
B	Serum anti-Müllerian hormone (AMH)
C	Serum CA125
D	Serum follicle-stimulating hormone (FSH) on days 10–12 of cycle
E	Serum FSH on day 21 of cycle
F	Serum FSH on days 2–5 of cycle
G	Serum luteinising hormone (LH) on day 5 of cycle
H	Serum LH on day 14 of cycle
I	Serum LH on day 21 of cycle
J	Serum progesterone on day 14 of cycle
K	Serum progesterone on day 21 of cycle
L	Serum progesterone on day 28 of cycle
M	Serum prolactin
N	Serum testosterone
O	Thyroid function tests

For each of the following clinical scenarios, what is the most appropriate investigation option from the list above? Each option may be used once, more than once or not at all.

362. A woman with a regular 35-day cycle attends the fertility clinic. Investigations are instigated. Which test should be arranged to check for ovulation?

363. Which test is probably the best biochemical marker of polycystic ovaries?

364. A 28-year-old woman with a BMI of 21 kg/m² attends the fertility clinic with her partner. She has very infrequent periods. She is treated with clomifene therapy to induce ovulation, but the treatment fails. Which test will indicate if this woman is likely to have a good clinical and endocrine response to laparoscopic ovarian drilling?

Options for questions 365–367

A	Abdominal examination
B	Abdominal ultrasound scan
C	Barium enema
D	Colonoscopy
E	CT scan of pelvis
F	Diagnostic laparoscopy
G	Diagnostic laparoscopy and peritoneal biopsy
H	Endoanal ultrasound
I	Endometrial biopsy
J	Endometrial cytokine levels
K	MRI of pelvis
L	Rectal examination
M	Serum CA125
N	Transperineal ultrasound scan
O	Transvaginal ultrasound scan
P	Vaginal examination

For each of the following clinical scenarios, what is the most appropriate management option from the list above? Each option may be used once, more than once or not at all.

365. A 35-year-old woman presents to the gynaecology clinic with pelvic pain and dysmenorrhoea. A pelvic examination demonstrates tenderness and fullness in the right iliac fossa. Which test should be used to diagnose or exclude an ovarian endometrioma?

366. A 24-year-old woman, *virgo intacta*, presents to the gynaecology clinic with abdominal and pelvic pain, dysmenorrhoea and dyschezia. What is the most appropriate initial assessment for the diagnosis of endometriosis?

367. A woman with a previous diagnosis of pelvic endometriosis presents to the clinic with cylical rectal bleeding. Vaginal and rectal examinations are inconclusive. What is the most appropriate initial assessment to identify or exclude rectal endometriosis?

Options for questions 368–370

A	Anabolic steroid abuse
B	Congenital bilateral absence of vas deferens (CBAVD)
C	Idiopathic
D	Kallmann syndrome
E	Kartagener's syndrome
F	Klinefelter syndrome
G	Maturation arrest
H	Noonan syndrome
I	Pituitary adenoma
J	Primary testicular failure
K	Retrograde ejaculation
L	Seminoma
M	Sertoli cell-only syndrome
N	Varicocele
O	Vasectomy
P	Y chromosome microdeletion

For each of the following clinical scenarios, what is the most likely diagnosis from the options listed? Each option may be used once, more than once or not at all.

368. A man is found to have azoospermia during the course of fertility investigations. He has two children from a previous relationship. He denies any significant medical history. On examination, he is muscular and both testes are small and soft.

369. A man is found to have azoospermia. His serum FSH and testosterone levels are normal. On examination, he has normal secondary sexual characteristics and both testes are of normal size. His karyotype is normal and a cystic fibrosis screen is negative. A testicular biopsy shows germ cells to be present.

370. A man is found to have azoospermia. His serum FSH level is elevated but his testosterone is normal. On examination, the man is tall and has gynaecomastia. Both testes are in the scrotum but are small and soft.

Answers

SBAs

341. Answer **D** 6 months

Explanation
Conception should be delayed for 6 months after radioactive iodine therapy.

Reference

Jefferys A, Vanderpump M, Yasmin E. Thyroid dysfunction and reproductive health. *The Obstetrician & Gynaecologist* 2015;17:39–45.

342. Answer **A** Idiopathic

Explanation
Causes of testicular failure include bilateral cryptorchidism, genetic disorders, systemic disease, radiotherapy and chemotherapy. However, in the majority of cases (66%), the cause is unknown.

Reference

Karavolos S, Stewart J, Evbuomwan I, McEleny K, Aird I. Assessment of the infertile male. *The Obstetrician & Gynaecologist* 2013;15:1–9.

343. Answer **B** 25%

Explanation
The main causes of infertility in the UK are (percentage figures indicate approximate prevalence):

- Unexplained infertility (no identified male or female cause): 25%
- Ovulatory disorders: 25%
- Tubal damage: 20%
- Factors in the male causing infertility: 30%
- Uterine or peritoneal disorders: 10%.

Reference

NICE. Fertility problems: assessment and treatment. *NICE Guidance (CG 156)*. Updated September 2017.

344. Answer **A** Female age

Explanation
A woman's age remains the single most important factor in determining reproductive outcome; ovarian reserve can only predict ovarian response in an assisted reproductive technology cycle.

Reference

Nandi A, Homburg R. Unexplained subfertility: diagnosis and management. *The Obstetrician & Gynaecologist* 2016;18:107–15.

345. Answer **A** Basal FSH in the early follicular phase

Explanation
Although the basal FSH test is the most frequently used, it has significant intra- and intercycle variability, which limits its reliability.

Reference

Nandi A, Homburg R. Unexplained subfertility: diagnosis and management. *The Obstetrician & Gynaecologist* 2016;18:107–15.

346. Answer **B** Explain that there is no known association between adenomyosis and subfertility

Explanation
The impact of adenomyosis or its treatment on fertility remains unsubstantiated because of a paucity of data. Therefore, subfertility in women with adenomyosis currently remains unexplained.

Reference

Nandi A, Homburg R. Unexplained subfertility: diagnosis and management. *The Obstetrician & Gynaecologist* 2016;18:107–15.

347. Answer **A** Conservative management

Explanation
There is insufficient evidence that myomectomy for intramural or subserous fibroids improves pregnancy rates.

Reference

Nandi A, Homburg R. Unexplained subfertility: diagnosis and management. *The Obstetrician & Gynaecologist* 2016;18:107–15.

348. Answer **E** Spontaneous intrauterine pregnancy

Explanation
Assessment of tubal patency can be achieved by various methods, such as HSG, HyCoSy, and laparoscopy and dye tests. None of these methods, however, can detect tubal function defects, which can potentially contribute to a couple's subfertility.
    If a couple conceive spontaneously and the pregnancy is intrauterine, then the fallopian tube must be functioning correctly.

Reference

Nandi A, Homburg R. Unexplained subfertility: diagnosis and management. *The Obstetrician & Gynaecologist* 2016;18:107–15.

349. Answer **D** Spermatid

Explanation
Sperm are formed in the seminiferous tubules, from germinal cells called spermatogonia. Spermatogonia divide by mitosis into primary spermatocytes, which in turn undergo two reduction divisions (meiosis I and II) to form spermatids.

Reference

Karavolos S, Stewart J, Evbuomwan I, McEleny K, Aird I. Assessment of the infertile male. *The Obstetrician & Gynaecologist* 2013;15:1–9.

350. Answer **B** 30%

Explanation
Long-term data from the Human Fertilisation and Embryology Authority (HFEA) analysing male factors as a cause for referral to fertility centres have shown that the percentage of infertility attributable to male factors appears to have increased from 27.6% in 2000 to 32.5% in 2006, but since then has averaged approximately 30%.

Reference

Karavolos S, Stewart J, Evbuomwan I, McEleny K, Aird I. Assessment of the infertile male. *The Obstetrician & Gynaecologist* 2013;15:1–9.

351. Answer **D** Only cases of severe and critical OHSS

Explanation
Licensed centres should comply with HFEA regulations in reporting cases of severe or critical OHSS among their patients.

Reference

RCOG. The management of ovarian hyperstimulation syndrome. *RCOG GTG No. 5.* February 2016.

352. Answer **B** Ibuprofen

Explanation
Relief of abdominal pain and nausea forms an important part of the supportive care of women with OHSS. Analgesia with paracetamol and opiates, if required, is appropriate, while non-steroidal anti-inflammatory drugs (NSAIDs) should be avoided as they may compromise renal function.

Reference

RCOG. The management of ovarian hyperstimulation syndrome. *RCOG GTG No. 5.* February 2016.

353. Answer **B** Mild OHSS

Explanation
See Table 3 in the reference article.

Reference

RCOG. The management of ovarian hyperstimulation syndrome. *RCOG GTG No. 5.* February 2016.

354. Answer **B** Laparoscopic salpingectomy

Explanation
Women with hydrosalpinges should be offered salpingectomy, preferably by laparoscopy, before IVF treatment because this improves the chance of a live birth.

Reference

NICE. Fertility problems: assessment and treatment. *NICE Guidance (CG 156).* Updated September 2017.

355. Answer **C** 7 days prior to the onset of menstruation, immediately before the start of ovarian stimulation

Explanation
The conclusions of studies to date suggest that an endometrial scratch should be carried out approximately 7 days prior to the onset of menstruation, immediately before the start of ovarian stimulation for IVF treatment.

Reference

RCOG. Local endometrial trauma (endometrial scratch): a treatment strategy to improve implantation rates. *RCOG Scientific Impact Paper No. 54.* November 2016.

EMQs

356. Answer **E** ICSI with donated eggs

Explanation
The woman is >45 years and appears to be perimenopausal. It is very unlikely that she would respond to ovarian stimulation. Even if eggs were retrieved, her chance of a successful pregnancy would be around 3% (HFEA data). With donated eggs, her chance of pregnancy would be around 50%. The semen analysis is very suboptimal, so ICSI is almost certainly required.

357. Answer **M** Ovulation induction and donor intrauterine insemination

Explanation
The female clinical picture is that of polycystic ovarian syndrome (PCOS). With an irregular cycle, she is unlikely to be ovulating consistently and therefore ovulation induction is required.

The male has maturation arrest, and therefore donor sperm will be required as it is not possible to use immature gametes for treatment in the UK.

358. Answer **K** No treatment required

Explanation
This couple have unexplained infertility, despite the history of orchidopexy. As the woman is <35 years and they have been trying to conceive for <2 years, no treatment is required at this moment in time. If they have still not conceived after 2 years, then the recommended treatment would be IVF.

Reference
NICE. Fertility problems: assessment and treatment. *NICE Guideline (CG156)*. Updated September 2017.

359. Answer **P** Weight loss

Explanation
Advise women with World Health Organization (WHO) group II anovulatory infertility who have a BMI of $\geq$30 kg/m^2 to lose weight. Inform them that this alone may restore ovulation, improve their response to ovulation induction agents and have a positive impact on pregnancy outcomes.

360. Answer **J** No treatment required

Explanation
Do not offer oral ovarian stimulation agents (such as clomifene citrate, anastrozole or letrozole) to women with unexplained infertility.

361. Answer **G** Laparoscopic ovarian drilling

Explanation
For women with WHO group II ovulation disorders who are known to be resistant to clomifene citrate, consider one of the following second-line treatments, depending on clinical circumstances and the woman's preference:

- Laparoscopic ovarian drilling
- Combined treatment with clomifene citrate and metformin if not already offered as a first-line treatment
- Gonadotropins.

In this case, the woman's symptoms could be suggestive of endometriosis, so laparoscopic ovarian drilling would allow inspection of the peritoneal cavity at the same time.

Reference
NICE. Fertility problems: assessment and treatment. *NICE Guideline (CG156)*. Updated September 2017.

362. Answer **L** Serum progesterone on day 28 of her cycle

Explanation
Serum progesterone should be measured 7 days before the expected day of menstruation.

363. Answer **B** Serum AMH

Explanation
It has been suggested recently that the threshold number of follicles to define a polycystic ovary should be 25, and that the biochemical marker of AMH may be even more precise than ultrasound, with a threshold serum concentration of >35 pmol/l.

364. Answer **G** Serum LH on day 5 of her cycle

Explanation
After laparoscopic ovarian drilling, with restoration of ovarian activity, serum concentrations of LH and testosterone fall. The response depends on pretreatment characteristics, with those who are slim and with high basal LH concentrations having a better clinical and endocrine response.

Reference

Balen AH. Polycystic ovary syndrome (PCOS). *The Obstetrician & Gynaecologist* 2017;19:119–29.

365. Answer **O** Transvaginal ultrasound scan

Explanation
Clinicians are recommended to perform transvaginal sonography to diagnose or to exclude ovarian endometrioma.

366. Answer **L** Rectal examination

Explanation
The guideline development group recommends that clinicians perform a clinical examination in all women with suspected endometriosis, although vaginal examination may be inappropriate for adolescents and/or women without previous sexual intercourse. In such cases, a rectal examination can be helpful for the diagnosis of endometriosis.

367. Answer **O** Transvaginal ultrasound scan

Explanation
In women with symptoms and signs of rectal endometriosis, transvaginal sonography is useful for identifying or ruling out rectal endometriosis.

Reference

ESHRE. Management of women with endometriosis. *ESHRE Guideline*. September 2013.

368 Answer **A** Anabolic steroid abuse

Explanation
The man already has children so has proven fertility. This rules out many of the causes of azoospermia above. Anabolic steroid abuse is common in gym users and results in pituitary suppression. This is the most likely cause of his azoospermia and small testes.

369. Answer   **G**   Maturation arrest

Explanation

With maturation arrest, germ cells are present in the testes, but the process of spermatogenesis is arrested, at either the spermatocyte or spermatid stage. This will result in azoospermia, but a testicular biopsy will confirm germ cells to be present. Leydig and Sertoli cells are present so there will be normal secondary sexual characteristics and normal feedback to the pituitary, resulting in a normal serum FSH.

370. Answer   **F**   Klinefelter syndrome

Explanation

From the clinical description, this is most likely to be Klinefelter's syndrome (karyotype 47,XXY), which can be confirmed by karyotyping. Primary testicular failure is also possible, but the features of a tall man with gynaecomastia make it much more likely that this is a case of Klinefelter syndrome.

Reference

Karavolos S, Stewart J, Evbuomwan I, McEleny K, Aird I. Assessment of the infertile male. *The Obstetrician & Gynaecologist* 2013;15:1–9.

Sexual and reproductive health

SBAs

371. Spasm of which muscle of the pelvic floor is most commonly implicated in vaginismus?

    A. Coccygeus
    B. Iliococcygeus
    C. Obturator internus
    D. Piriformis
    E. Pubococcygeus

372. What is the most common cause of hypoactive sexual desire disorder (HSDD)?

    A. Depression
    B. Drug-induced
    C. Menopause
    D. Psychosexual
    E. Surgically induced

373. Which method of emergency contraception works primarily by inhibiting fertilisation?

    A. Copper intrauterine contraceptive device (IUCD)
    B. Levonorgestrel-releasing intrauterine system (LNG-IUS)
    C. Oral levonorgestrel
    D. Ulipristal acetate
    E. Yuzpe regimem

374. According to the *UK Medical Eligibility Criteria for Contraceptive Use* (UKMEC), what is the medical contraindication to the use of levonorgestrel for emergency contraception?

    A. Breastfeeding
    B. Female age >35 years
    C. No medical contraindications
    D. Nulliparity
    E. Previous ectopic pregnancy

375. What is the failure rate of the lactational amenorrhoea method (LAM) of postpartum contraception?
    A. 2 in 100 women
    B. 2 in 500 women
    C. 2 in 1000 women
    D. 2 in 5000 women
    E. 2 in 10,000 women

376. Once a menopausal woman is established on hormone replacement therapy (HRT), how often should she be reviewed?
    A. 3-monthly
    B. 6-monthly
    C. Annually
    D. Every 2 years
    E. Every 5 years

377. What is the most sensitive test for detection of *Trichomonas vaginalis* infection?
    A. Immunochromatographic capillary flow (dipstick) assay
    B. Laboratory culture
    C. Light-field microscopy
    D. Nucleic acid amplification test (NAAT)
    E. *Trichomonas* serum antibody test

378. A 47-year-old woman who has been using condoms for contraception with her partner attends for contraceptive advice. Her last menstrual period was 8 months ago and she has no overt menopausal symptoms.

    Assuming she has no further periods, for how long should she continue to use contraception?
    A. She can stop now as the chances of conception are so low
    B. 4 months
    C. 12 months
    D. 16 months
    E. 24 months

379. Which two hormonal methods of contraception are associated with the highest failure rate in perimenopausal women in the first year of typical (non-perfect) use?

	Combined hormonal contraception	LNG-IUS	Progestogen-only implant	Progestogen-only injectable	Progestogen-only pill
A	✓	✓			
B		✓	✓		
C			✓	✓	
D				✓	✓
E	✓				✓

380. *Chlamydia trachomatis* infection is known to have a high frequency of transmission.

If one partner is infected, what is the likelihood that the other partner will also be infected?

A. 10%
B. 25%
C. 50%
D. 75%
E. 100%

EMQs

Options for questions 381–384

A	Aciclovir 400 mg orally three times per day for 21 days
B	Azithromycin 1 g orally as a single dose
C	Ceftriaxone 500 mg intramuscularly plus azithromycin 1 g orally
D	Clindamycin orally 300 mg twice daily for 7 days
E	Clotrimazole vaginal pessary 1 g for 5 nights
F	Fluconazole 1 g orally
G	Fluconazole 150 mg every 72 hours for three doses
H	Metronidazole 2 g orally as a single dose
I	Metronidazole 500 mg orally twice daily for 14 days
J	Nevirapine intravenous stat dose
K	Ofloxacin 400 mg twice daily orally plus oral metronidazole 400 mg twice daily for 14 days
L	Valaciclovir 500 mg twice daily for 5 days
M	Zidovudine intravenous infusion

Each of the following clinical scenarios relates to a woman with a pelvic infection. For each woman, select the single most appropriate initial management from the list above. Each option may be used once, more than once or not at all.

381. A 26-year-old woman attends the gynaecology emergency services complaining of painful blisters and ulceration on her vulva for last 2 days. She has dysuria and vaginal discharge. On examination, there is bilateral tender inguinal lymphadenitis.

382. A 21-year-old woman who suffers with alcohol dependence attends the gynaecology clinic complaining of a persistent watery vaginal discharge. There is no history of irritation or pruritus. She smokes ten cigarettes a day. On vaginal examination, there is an offensive fishy-smelling vaginal discharge.

383. A 23-year-old university student complains of persistent purulent vaginal discharge. On vaginal examination, there is contact bleeding from the cervix. Microscopy of a Gram-stained endocervical swab specimen showed monomorphic Gram-negative diplococci within polymorphonuclear leucocytes.

384. A 49-year-old menopausal diabetic woman presents with vulval soreness and pruritus, and a non-offensive thick white vaginal discharge. She gives a history of at least three past similar episodes over the last 12 months and suffers from superficial dyspareunia. On examination, there is erythema and some fissuring of the vulval skin.

Options for questions 385–387

A	Black cohosh
B	Clonidine
C	Cognitive behavioural therapy (CBT)
D	Oestradiol implant
E	Oestriol cream vaginally
F	Oral conjugated equine oestrogens
G	Oral continuous combined HRT
H	Oral cyclical HRT
I	Oral oestradiol
J	Psychosexual counselling
K	St John's wort
L	Testosterone gel
M	Testosterone implant
N	Tibolone
O	Transdermal continuous combined HRT
P	Transdermal cyclical HRT
Q	Transdermal oestrogen

For each of the following clinical scenarios, choose the single most appropriate treatment from the list of options above. Each option may be used once, more than once or not at all.

385. A 52-year-old woman with a BMI of 31 kg/m^2 presents with vasomotor symptoms and vaginal dryness. She has no significant past medical history. Her last menstrual period was 12 months ago.

386. A 50-year-old woman who previously had a hysterectomy for uterine fibroids presents with severe menopausal symptoms. She is concerned about taking HRT as her elder sister recently had a stroke.

387. A 54-year-old woman who is taking continuous combined HRT presents with a lack of libido.

Options for questions 388–390

A	*Candida albicans*
B	*Chlamydia trachomatis*
C	*Gardnerella vaginalis*
D	*Haemophilus ducreyi*
E	Herpes simplex virus
F	Herpes zoster virus
G	Human papillomavirus
H	Molluscum contagiosum virus
I	*Mycoplasma genitalium*
J	*Neisseria gonorrhoeae*
K	*Phthirus pubis*
L	*Sarcoptes scabiei*
M	*Treponema pallidum*
N	*Trichomonas vaginalis*

In each of the following scenarios, what is the most likely organism that is being described? Each option may be used once, more than once or not at all.

388. A large DNA pox virus that causes a benign epidermal eruption of the skin. The lesions are usually characteristic, presenting as smooth-surfaced, firm, dome-shaped papules with central umbilication.

389. A sexually transmitted infection commonly presenting with vulval discharge and itching, dysuria and offensive odour. Overall, 10–50% of women are asymptomatic. Of women that are infected, the urethra is colonised in 90%, and 2% of women will have a 'strawberry cervix'.

390. Permethrin is the first-line treatment for infection with this organism. Classic sites of infection include the interdigital folds, the wrists and elbows, and around the nipples in women.

Answers

SBAs

371. Answer   **E**   Pubococcygeus

Explanation
Vaginismus is the involuntary spasm of the pubococcygeal and associated muscles causing painful and difficult penetration of the vagina during intercourse, tampon insertion or clinical examination.

Reference

Cowan F, Frodsham L. Management of common disorders in psychosexual medicine. *The Obstetrician & Gynaecologist* 2015;17:47–53.

372. Answer   **D**   Psychosexual

Explanation
Most patients with HSDD will have a psychosexual cause but organic causes can include menopause, depression, drug therapy such as selective serotonin reuptake inhibitors and tricyclic antidepressants, or it may be acquired, for example after bilateral oophrectomy, chemotherapy and irradiation.

Reference

Cowan F, Frodsham L. Management of common disorders in psychosexual medicine. *The Obstetrician & Gynaecologist* 2015;17:47–53.

373. Answer   **A**   Copper intrauterine contraceptive device (IUCD)

Explanation
Copper is toxic to the ovum and sperm, and thus a copper-bearing IUCD is effective immediately after insertion and works primarily by inhibiting fertilisation.

Reference

FSRH. Emergency contraception. *FSRH Guideline*. Updated December 2017.

374. Answer   **C**   No medical contraindications

Explanation
UKMEC advises that there are no medical contraindications to levonorgestrel, including breastfeeding.

Reference

FSRH. Emergency contraception. *FSRH Guideline*. Updated December 2017.

375. Answer   **A**   2 in 100 women

Explanation
LAM is a temporary contraceptive method that relies on exclusive breastfeeding. It has a failure rate of around 2 in 100 women.

Reference

RCOG. Postpartum family planning. *RCOG Best Practice Paper No. 1*. June 2015.

376. **Answer**   **C**   Annually

    Explanation
    Once established on HRT, an annual review is all that is necessary. HRT does not increase blood pressure and there is no indication to monitor more frequently.

    Reference

    Bakour SH, Williamson J. Latest evidence on using hormone replacement therapy in the menopause. *The Obstetrician & Gynaecologist* 2015;17:20–8.

377. **Answer**   **D**   Nucleic acid amplification test (NAAT)

    Explanation
    NAATs offer the highest sensitivity for the detection of *T. vaginalis*. They should be the test of choice where resources allow and are becoming the current 'gold standard'. In-house polymerase chain reaction (PCR) tests have shown increased sensitivity in comparison with both microscopy and culture.

    Reference

    Sherrard J, Ison C, Moody J, *et al.* United Kingdom national guideline on the management of *Trichomonas vaginalis*. *International Journal of STD & AIDS* 2014;25:541–9.

378. **Answer**   **D**   16 months

    Explanation
    For women over the age of 50 who do not use hormonal methods, contraception can be stopped after 1 year of amenorrhoea as fertility is unlikely to return. In women <50 years, contraception should be continued for 2 years, as the return of fertile ovulation is more likely to occur.

    Reference

    Bakour SH, Hatti A, Whalen S. Contraceptive methods and issues around the menopause: an evidence update. *The Obstetrician & Gynaecologist* 2017;19:289–97.

379. **Answer**   **E**   Combined hormonal contraception and progestogen-only pill

    Explanation
    See Table 1 in the reference article.

    Reference

    Bakour SH, Hatti A, Whalen S. Contraceptive methods and issues around the menopause: an evidence update. *The Obstetrician & Gynaecologist* 2017;19:289–97.

380. **Answer**   **D**   75%

    Explanation
    Chlamydia infection has a high frequency of transmission, with concordance rates of up to 75% of partners being reported.

    Reference

    Nwokolo NC, Dragovic B, Patel S, *et al.* 2015 UK national guideline for the management of infection with *Chlamydia trachomatis*. *International Journal of STD & AIDS* 2016;27:251–67.

EMQs

381. Answer   L   Valaciclovir 500 mg twice daily for 5 days

Explanation

The woman has genital herpes. The other possible medication used to treat anogenital herpes is aciclovir, but the doses described in the list of options are incorrect.

Reference

Patel R, Green J, Clarke E, *et al.* 2014 UK national guideline for the management of anogenital herpes. *International Journal of STD & AIDS* 2015;26:763–76.

382. Answer   D   Clindamycin orally 300 mg twice daily for 7 days

Explanation

The clinical features are typical of bacterial vaginosis and the other treatments mentioned in the list are not applicable for bacterial vaginosis. The doses of metronidazole are incorrect. Both oral and topical metronidazole should not be used if alcohol cannot be avoided.

Reference

BASHH. UK national guideline for the management of bacterial vaginosis. *Clinical Effectiveness Group, British Association for Sexual Health and HIV*. Updated 2012.

383. Answer   C   Ceftriaxone 500 mg intramuscularly plus azithromycin 1 g orally

Explanation

The clinical features and laboratory findings are typical of gonococcal infection. Ofloxacin and moxifloxacin should be avoided in patients who are at high risk of gonococcal pelvic inflammatory disease (PID) (e.g. when the patient's partner has gonorrhoea, in clinically severe disease or following sexual contact abroad), because of increasing quinolone resistance in the UK. Quinolones should also be avoided as the first-line empirical treatment for PID in areas where >5% of PID is caused by quinolone-resistant *Neisseria gonorrhoeae*.

Reference

Bignell C, Fitzgerald M on behalf of BASHH. UK national guideline for the management of gonorrhoea in adults, 2011. *International Journal of STD & AIDS* 2011;22:541–7.

384. Answer   G   Fluconazole 150 mg every 72 hours for three doses

Explanation

This woman has typical history and features of recurrent vulvovaginal candidiasis. The other treatments mentioned are not applicable for recurrent candida infection.

Reference

BASHH. United Kingdom national guideline on the management of vulvovaginal candidiasis. *BASHH Guideline*. June 2007.

385. Answer   **O**   Transdermal continuous combined HRT

Explanation
Consider transdermal rather than oral HRT for menopausal women who are at increased risk of previous venous thromboembolism (VTE), including those with a BMI >30 kg/m².

386. Answer   **Q**   Transdermal oestrogen

Explanation
Explain to women that taking oral (but not transdermal) oestrogen is associated with a small increase in the risk of stroke. Also explain that the baseline population risk of stroke in women aged <60 years is very low.

387. Answer   **L**   Testosterone gel

Explanation
Consider testosterone supplementation for menopausal women with low sexual desire if HRT alone is not effective.

Reference

NICE. Menopause: diagnosis and management. *NICE Guideline (NG23)*. November 2015.

388. Answer   **H**   Molluscum contagiosum virus

Reference

Fernando I, Pritchard J, Edwards SK, Grover D. UK national guideline for the management of genital molluscum in adults. *International Journal of STD & AIDS* 2015;26:687–95.

389. Answer   **N**   *Trichomonas vaginalis*

Reference

Sherrard J, Ison C, Moody J, *et al*. United Kingdom national guideline on the management of *Trichomonas vaginalis*. *International Journal of STD & AIDS* 2014;25:541–9.

390. Answer   **L**   *Sarcoptes scabiei*

Reference

BASHH. 2016 UK national guideline on the management of scabies. *BASHH Guideline*. March 2016.

Early pregnancy care

SBAs

391. What is the diagnostic tool of choice for tubal ectopic pregnancy?

    A. Laparoscopy
    B. MRI of pelvis
    C. Serial β-human chorionic gonadotropin (β-hCG) measurements
    D. Transabdominal ultrasound
    E. Transvaginal ultrasound

392. What proportion of ectopic pregnancies occur in the interstitial portion of the fallopian tube?

    A. 1–6%
    B. 7–10%
    C. 11–16%
    D. 17–20%
    E. 21–26%

393. A woman attends the early pregnancy unit having experienced some discomfort and vaginal bleeding in early pregnancy. It is 6 weeks since her last menstrual period. She is actively trying to conceive. A transvaginal ultrasound scan is performed, but there is no evidence of an intrauterine gestation sac. Her serum β-hCG level is 1200 IU/l. The β-hCG is repeated after 48 hours and is 950 IU/l.
    What is the most appropriate management?

    A. Diagnostic laparoscopy
    B. Discharge the patient
    C. Medical therapy with methotrexate
    D. Perform a urinary pregnancy test in 2–3 weeks
    E. Repeat a further β-hCG in 48 hours

394. A woman attends the early pregnancy unit with a small amount of per vaginam spotting. It is 7 weeks since her last menstrual period, but her cycle is irregular. A transvaginal scan is performed, which shows an intrauterine gestation sac measuring 15 mm in diameter. A follow-up scan is arranged 14 days later, which shows a gestation sac with a diameter of 24 mm. There is now a yolk sac visible with a fetal pole with a crown–rump length of 7 mm, but no fetal heartbeat is visible.

     What is the diagnosis?

     A. Incomplete miscarriage
     B. Missed miscarriage
     C. Pregnancy of unknown location
     D. Pregnancy of unknown viability
     E. Viable intrauterine pregnancy

395. What proportion of miscarriages occur after the identification of fetal heart activity?

     A. <5%
     B. 5–8%
     C. 9–12%
     D. 13–17%
     E. 18–24%

396. Which objective and validated index is typically used to classify the severity of nausea and vomiting in pregnancy (NVP)?

     A. Morning sickness evaluation score
     B. Korttila scale
     C. Pregnancy-unique quantification of emesis (PUQE)
     D. Rhodes index of nausea, vomiting and retching
     E. Value of eMesis score (VOMS)

397. At what gestation do the symptoms of NVP typically peak?

     A. 4 weeks
     B. 7 weeks
     C. 9 weeks
     D. 12 weeks
     E. 15 weeks

398. Which abnormality of acid–base balance is most commonly seen in women with NVP?

     A. Metabolic acidosis
     B. Metabolic acidosis with respiratory compensation
     C. Metabolic alkalosis
     D. Respiratory acidosis
     E. Respiratory alkalosis

399. What is the most appropriate solution for intravenous rehydration in women with NVP?

   A. 5% dextrose
   B. Hartmann's solution
   C. Human albumin solution 4%
   D. Normal saline 0.9%
   E. Normal saline 0.9% with potassium chloride

400. What triad of findings defines hyperemesis gravidarum in women with severe protracted NVP?

	Electrolyte imbalance	2% weight loss from prepregnancy	5% weight loss from prepregnancy	Dehydration	Ketonuria
A	✓	✓			✓
B	✓		✓	✓	
C		✓		✓	✓
D			✓	✓	✓
E	✓	✓		✓	

401. What proportion of women with hyperemesis gravidarum have abnormal thyroid function tests?

   A. 10%
   B. 33%
   C. 50%
   D. 66%
   E. 90%

402. A 25-year-old woman with no live births attends the recurrent miscarriage clinic. She has had three first-trimester miscarriages in the past. During consultation, she enquires about her chances of a successful pregnancy when she next becomes pregnant.
   Which figure should be quoted?

   A. 20%
   B. 40%
   C. 60%
   D. 80%
   E. 100%

403. What proportion of parents with recurrent miscarriage will be found to have a balanced chromosomal translocation if peripheral blood karyotyping is performed?

    A. 2%
    B. 12%
    C. 22%
    D. 32%
    E. 42%

404. What is the most common symptom in women who develop gestational trophoblastic disease after a miscarriage?

    A. Breast engorgement
    B. Nausea and vomiting
    C. Passing tissue vaginally
    D. Symptoms of hyperthyroidism
    E. Vaginal bleeding

405. A woman who is rhesus negative is diagnosed with a molar pregnancy and undergoes surgical evacuation of the uterus. Histological analysis confirms this to be a complete molar pregnancy.

    In terms of anti-D prophylaxis, what is the most appropriate management?

    A. Administer 250 IU anti-D
    B. Administer 1500 IU anti-D
    C. Anti-D is not required
    D. Arrange paternal genetic testing
    E. Perform a Kleihauer test

EMQs

Options for questions 406–408

A	Dilute Russell viper venom test
B	Glucose tolerance test
C	Karyotyping of products of conception
D	No test required
E	Ovarian autoantibodies
F	Parental peripheral blood karyotyping
G	Pelvic ultrasound scan
H	Peripheral blood natural killer cell testing
I	Serum cytokine levels
J	Thrombophilia screen
K	Thyroid function tests
L	Thyroid peroxidase antibodies
M	TORCH (toxoplasmosis, rubella virus, cytomegalovirus, herpes simplex virus and HIV) screen
N	Uterine natural killer cell testing

For each of the following clinical scenarios, choose the single next most appropriate test from the options listed. Each option may be used once, more than once or not at all.

406. A 32-year-old woman attends the miscarriage clinic for a follow-up appointment. She has previously been investigated for three recurrent first-trimester losses (all tests according to RCOG guidance), but now presents with a further pregnancy loss at 16 weeks of gestation.

407. A woman attends the miscarriage clinic after three consecutive miscarriages. All investigations are normal. She subsequently has a fourth miscarriage, which is managed surgically.

408. A 38-year-old woman is referred by her GP to the miscarriage clinic after two consecutive miscarriages.

Options for questions 409–411

A	Clinical examination
B	CT scan
C	Hysteroscopy
D	Laparoscopy
E	Laparotomy
F	MRI scan
G	No diagnostic test required
H	Serum α-fetoprotein (AFP)
I	Serum β-human chorionic gonadotropin (β-hCG)
J	Serum progesterone
K	Transabdominal ultrasound scan
L	Transperineal ultrasound
M	Transvaginal ultrasound scan

For each of the following scenarios, what is the most appropriate investigation from the options listed? Each option may be used once, more than once or not at all.

409. A 35-year-old woman who has had three previous caesarean sections presents with scar pain and vaginal bleeding at 7 weeks of gestation. What is the primary diagnostic modality for diagnosing caesarean scar pregnancies?

410. A 33-year-old woman in her fourth pregnancy is referred to an obstetric consultant following a late booking scan. It is 16 weeks since her last menstrual period. An ultrasound scan had shown an empty uterus but a gestation sac outside the uterus surrounded by loops of bowel. What diagnostic modality can be a useful adjunct in advanced abdominal pregnancy?

411. A 29-year-old woman attends the early pregnancy unit following in vitro fertilisation (IVF) treatment. She has mild abdominal tenderness and a small amount of vaginal bleeding. Her embryo transfer was 5 weeks previously and her pregnancy test is positive. The patient underwent IVF treatment due to tubal disease secondary to *Chlamydia* infection. What would be the diagnostic tool of choice for ectopic pregnancy in this situation?

Options for questions 412–414

A	Cornual resection
B	Dilation and curettage
C	Evacuation of retained products of conception
D	Expectant management
E	Hysteroscopic resection
F	Intramuscular methotrexate
G	Laparoscopic salpingectomy
H	Laparoscopic salpingotomy
I	Laparoscopy and proceed
J	Laparotomy and proceed
K	Manual vacuum aspiration
L	No treatment required
M	Potassium injected into the pregnancy under ultrasound guidance
N	Uterine artery embolisation

For each of the following scenarios, what is the most appropriate management from the options listed? Each option may be used once, more than once or not at all.

412. A woman presents to the early pregnancy unit with pain and bleeding at 6 weeks of gestation. An ultrasound scan is performed, which shows an empty uterus with a barrel-shaped cervix. There is a gestation sac below the level of the internal os with blood flow around the sac visible using colour Doppler.

413. A woman with a history of left ectopic pregnancy managed by salpingotomy attends the early pregnancy unit with right-sided pain and vaginal bleeding. It is 7 weeks since her last menstrual period. A transvaginal ultrasound scan demonstrates a mass in the right adnexa, which is tender. Her serum β-hCG level is 7800 IU/l.

414. A woman with a previous history of ectopic pregnancy attends the early pregnancy unit for a reassurance scan at 7 weeks of gestation. She has no symptoms. A transvaginal scan shows an empty uterus but a 32 mm left adnexal cystic mass separate from the ovary. A yolk sac and fetal pole are seen, but there is no fetal heartbeat. There is no free fluid. Her serum β-hCG is 3500 IU/l. This is repeated 48 hours later and is 3800 IU/l.

Options for questions 415–417

A	23,X
B	23,Y
C	45,XO
D	46,XX
E	46,XY
F	47,XXO
G	47,XXX
H	47,XXY
I	47,XYY
J	69,XXX
K	69,XXY
L	69,XYY
M	69,YYY

For each of the following clinical scenarios, what is the most likely karyotype from the options listed? Each option may be used once, more than once or not at all.

415. A woman presents with hyperemesis and bleeding to the gynaecology assessment unit. An ultrasound scan suggests a complete molar pregnancy and this is confirmed following histopathological analysis of the evacuated products of conception.
   What is the karyotype of the sperm that fertilised the oocyte?

416. A woman attends for a routine dating scan at 12 weeks of gestation. This shows an enlarged placenta with cystic spaces and a small fetus. A surgical evacuation is performed, which confirms a partial molar pregnancy.
   What is the most likely karyotype?

417. A recent immigrant to the UK presents with shortness of breath, haemoptysis and vaginal bleeding. She describes a 'miscarriage' a few months earlier. A pregnancy test is strongly positive and an ultrasound scan shows a haemorrhagic cystic mass in the uterus. A chest X-ray shows multiple nodules in both lungs.
   What is the most likely karyotype of the tumour?

Options for questions 418–420

A	<1%
B	10%
C	25%
D	33%
E	40%
F	50%
G	66%
H	75%
I	80%
J	90%

For each of the following clinical scenarios, what is the closest risk of each event occurring from the options listed? Each option may be used once, more than once or not at all.

418. The proportion of partial moles that are triploid in origin.

419. The proportion of ectopic pregnancies that are cervical pregnancies.

420. The risk of miscarriage in a recognised pregnancy in a woman aged 35–39 years.

Answers
SBAs

391. Answer **E** Transvaginal ultrasound

Explanation
Transvaginal ultrasound is the diagnostic tool of choice for tubal ectopic pregnancy.

Reference
RCOG. Diagnosis and management of ectopic pregnancy. *RCOG GTG No. 21*. November 2016.

392. Answer **A** 1–6%

Explanation
Interstitial ectopic pregnancy is when implantation occurs in the interstitial portion of the fallopian tube and occurs in 1–6% of ectopic pregnancies.

Reference
Al-Memar M, Kirk E, Bourne T. The role of ultrasonography in the diagnosis and management of early pregnancy complications. *The Obstetrician & Gynaecologist* 2015;17:173–81.

393. Answer **D** Perform a urinary pregnancy test in 2–3 weeks

Explanation
See Figure 4 in the reference article.

Reference
Al-Memar M, Kirk E, Bourne T. The role of ultrasonography in the diagnosis and management of early pregnancy complications. *The Obstetrician & Gynaecologist* 2015;17:173–81.

394. Answer **B** Missed miscarriage

A common-sense approach to the diagnosis of miscarriage was proposed following a consensus conference of the US Society for Radiologists in Ultrasound in 2012. The authors proposed that on a follow-up transvaginal ultrasound scan, a diagnosis of pregnancy failure may be made on the basis of the following findings:

- An embryo with a crown–rump length of >7 mm with no heartbeat
- A mean gestational sac diameter of >25 mm with no embryo
- Absence of an embryo with a heartbeat if >2 weeks has elapsed following a scan that showed a gestational sac without a yolk sac
- Absence of an embryo with a heartbeat >11 days after a scan that showed a gestational sac and yolk sac.

Reference
Al-Memar M, Kirk E, Bourne T. The role of ultrasonography in the diagnosis and management of early pregnancy complications. *The Obstetrician & Gynaecologist* 2015;17:173–81.

395. Answer **A** <5%

Explanation
Less than 5% of miscarriages occur after the identification of fetal heart activity.

Reference

Saraswat L, Ashok PW, Mathur M. Medical management of miscarriage. *The Obstetrician & Gynaecologist* 2014;16:79–85.

396. Answer **C** Pregnancy-unique quantification of emesis (PUQE)

Explanation
An objective and validated index of nausea and vomiting such as the PUQE score can be used to classify the severity of NVP.

The Rhodes index was originally validated to measure nausea and vomiting in chemotherapy patients, including assessment of physical symptoms and the resulting stress, but has subsequently been used for NVP.

Reference

RCOG. The management of nausea and vomiting of pregnancy and hyperemesis gravidarum. *RCOG GTG No. 69.* June 2016.

397. Answer **C** 9 weeks

Explanation
NVP typically starts between 4 and 7 weeks of gestation, peaking at approximately week 9 and resolving by week 20 in 90% of women.

Reference

RCOG. The management of nausea and vomiting of pregnancy and hyperemesis gravidarum. *RCOG GTG No. 69.* June 2016.

398. Answer **C** Metabolic alkalosis

Explanation
NVP and hyperemesis gravidarum are associated with hyponatraemia, hypokalaemia, low serum urea, a raised haematocrit and ketonuria with a metabolic hypochloraemic alkalosis.

Reference

RCOG. The management of nausea and vomiting of pregnancy and hyperemesis gravidarum. *RCOG GTG No. 69.* June 2016.

399. Answer **E** Normal saline 0.9% with potassium chloride

Explanation
Normal saline with additional potassium chloride in each bag, with administration guided by daily monitoring of electrolytes, is the most appropriate method of intravenous hydration for NVP.

Reference

RCOG. The management of nausea and vomiting of pregnancy and hyperemesis gravidarum. *RCOG GTG No. 69.* June 2016.

400. Answer   **B**   Electrolyte imbalance, 5% weight loss from prepregnancy weight and dehydration

Explanation
Hyperemesis gravidarum is characterised by severe, protracted nausea and vomiting associated with weight loss of >5% of prepregnancy weight, dehydration and electrolyte imbalances.

Reference
RCOG. The management of nausea and vomiting of pregnancy and hyperemesis gravidarum. *RCOG GTG No. 69*. June 2016.

401. Answer   **D**   66%

Explanation
In two-thirds of patients with hyperemesis gravidarum, there may be abnormal thyroid function tests (based on a structural similarity between thyroid-stimulating hormone (TSH) and β-hCG) with a biochemical thyrotoxicosis and raised free thyroxine levels with or without a suppressed TSH level. These patients rarely have thyroid antibodies and are euthyroid clinically. The biochemical thyrotoxicosis resolves as the hyperemesis gravidarum improves, and treatment with antithyroid drugs is inappropriate.

Reference
RCOG. The management of nausea and vomiting of pregnancy and hyperemesis gravidarum. *RCOG GTG No. 69*. June 2016.

402. Answer   **C**   60%

Explanation
Previous reproductive history is an independent predictor of future pregnancy outcome. The risk of a further miscarriage increases after each successive pregnancy loss, reaching approximately 40% after three consecutive pregnancy losses, and the prognosis worsens with increasing maternal age.

Reference
RCOG. The investigation and treatment of couples with recurrent first trimester and second-trimester miscarriage. *RCOG GTG No. 17*. April 2011.

403. Answer   **A**   2%

Explanation
A recent retrospective UK audit of four UK centres over periods of 5–30 years reported that balanced translocations were found in 1.99% (406 out of 20,432) of parents with recurrent miscarriage.

Reference
RCOG. The investigation and treatment of couples with recurrent first trimester and second-trimester miscarriage. *RCOG GTG No. 17*. April 2011.

404. Answer **E** Vaginal bleeding

Explanation
Several case series have shown that vaginal bleeding is the most common presenting symptom of gestational trophoblastic disease diagnosed after miscarriage, therapeutic termination of pregnancy or postpartum.

Reference
RCOG. The management of gestational trophoblastic disease. *RCOG GTG No. 38*. March 2010.

405. Answer **C** Anti-D is not required

Explanation
Because of poor vascularisation of the chorionic villi and absence of the anti-D antigen in complete moles, anti-D prophylaxis is not required. It is, however, required for partial moles. Confirmation of the diagnosis of a complete molar pregnancy may not occur for some time after evacuation and so administration of anti-D could be delayed when required, within an appropriate timeframe.

Reference
RCOG. The management of gestational trophoblastic disease. *RCOG GTG No. 38*. March 2010.

EMQs

406. Answer **J** Thrombophilia screen

Explanation
Women with a second-trimester miscarriage should be screened for inherited thrombophilias including factor V Leiden, factor II (prothrombin) gene mutation and protein S.

407. Answer **C** Karyotyping of products of conception

Explanation
Cytogenetic analysis should be performed on the products of conception of the third and subsequent consecutive miscarriage(s).

408. Answer **D** No test required

Explanation
Recurrent miscarriage, defined as the loss of three or more consecutive pregnancies, affects 1% of couples trying to conceive. There is no need to investigate after two miscarriages.

Reference
RCOG. The investigation and treatment of couples with recurrent first trimester and second-trimester miscarriage. *RCOG GTG No. 17*. April 2011.

409. Answer   **M**   Transvaginal ultrasound scan

Explanation
Clinicians should be aware that ultrasound is the primary diagnostic modality, using a transvaginal approach, supplemented by transabdominal imaging if required.

410. Answer   **F**   MRI scan

Explanation
MRI can be a useful diagnostic adjunct in advanced abdominal pregnancy and can help to plan the surgical approach.

411. Answer   **M**   Transvaginal ultrasound scan

Explanation
A transvaginal ultrasound scan is the diagnostic tool of choice for tubal ectopic pregnancies.

Reference

RCOG. Diagnosis and management of ectopic pregnancy. *RCOG GTG No. 21*. November 2016.

412. Answer   **F**   Intramuscular methotrexate

Explanation
Medical management with methotrexate can be considered for cervical pregnancy. Surgical methods of management are associated with a high failure rate and should be reserved for those women suffering life-threatening bleeding.
    A retrospective review of 62 cases of cervical ectopic pregnancy estimated the efficacy of systemic methotrexate administration in the treatment of cervical ectopic pregnancy to be approximately 91%.

413. Answer   **H**   Laparoscopic salpingotomy

Explanation
A laparoscopic surgical approach is preferable to an open approach. In women with a history of fertility-reducing factors (previous ectopic pregnancy, contralateral tubal damage, previous abdominal surgery, previous pelvic inflammatory disease), salpingotomy should be considered.
    Success rates for methotrexate are only 38% if β-hCG levels are >5000 IU/l.

414. Answer   **F**   Intramuscular methotrexate

Explanation
NICE recommends that methotrexate should be the first-line management for women who are able to return for follow-up and who have:

- No significant pain
- An unruptured ectopic pregnancy with a mass smaller than 35 mm with no visible heartbeat

- A serum β-hCG between 1500 and 5000 IU/l
- No intrauterine pregnancy (as confirmed by an ultrasound scan).

Expectant management is not appropriate as the serum β-hCG level is rising.

Reference

RCOG. Diagnosis and management of ectopic pregnancy. *RCOG GTG No. 21*. November 2016.

415. Answer   **A**   23,X

Explanation

Complete moles usually (75–80%) arise as a consequence of duplication of a single sperm following fertilisation of an 'empty' ovum.

Two Y chromosomes are not compatible with development, so as duplication is the most likely cause, the sperm must have been 23X.

Reference

RCOG. The management of gestational trophoblastic disease. *RCOG GTG No. 38*. March 2010.

416. Answer   **K**   69,XXY

Explanation

The frequencies of the karyotypes of partial moles are:

69,XXY	70%
69,XXX	27%
69,XYY	3%

Reference

Nyberg DA, McGahan JP, Pretorius DH, Pilu G (eds.). *Diagnostic Imaging of Fetal Anomalies*. Philadelphia: Lippincott Williams & Wilkins, 2003.

417. Answer   **D**   46,XX

This is likely to be a choriocarcinoma, and 50% of these tumours arise from a hydatidiform mole. The majority (90%) of hydatidiform moles have the karyotype 46,XX.

Reference

Fox H, Buckley CH. *Pathology for Gynaecologists*. 2nd edn. London: Hodder Arnold, 1991.

418. Answer   **J**   90%

Explanation

Partial moles are usually (90%) triploid in origin, with two sets of paternal haploid genes and one set of maternal haploid genes.

Reference

RCOG. The management of gestational trophoblastic disease. *RCOG GTG No. 38*. March 2010.

419. Answer   **A**   <1%

Explanation
Cervical pregnancies are rare, accounting for <1% of all ectopic gestations.

Reference

RCOG. Diagnosis and management of ectopic pregnancy. *RCOG GTG No. 21*. November 2016.

420. Answer   **C**   25%

Explanation
The age-related risks of miscarriage in recognised pregnancies are:

12–19 years	13%
20–24 years	11%
25–29 years	12%
30–34 years	15%
35–39 years	25%
40–44 years	51%
≥45 years	93%

Reference

RCOG. The investigation and treatment of couples with recurrent first trimester and second-trimester miscarriage. *RCOG GTG No. 17*. April 2011.

Gynaecological oncology

SBAs

421. To which group of lymph nodes does a squamous cell carcinoma of the vulva initially spread?

   A. External iliac
   B. Femoral
   C. Inguinal
   D. Internal iliac
   E. Para-aortic

422. A 70-year-old woman presents with vulval itching and bleeding. On examination, a suspicious lesion is identified and an excision biopsy is performed. The lesion is confirmed as a squamous cell carcinoma with depth of invasion of <1 mm.
   What is the likelihood of lymph node involvement?

   A. <1%
   B. 5%
   C. 10%
   D. 15%
   E. 20%

423. Which two chemotherapeutic agents are most commonly used in the management of ovarian cancer?

	Carboplatin	Chlorambucil	Cisplatin	Cyclophosphamide	Paclitaxel
A	✓	✓			
B		✓	✓		
C			✓	✓	
D				✓	✓
E	✓				✓

424. From which type of tumour does a secondary tumour of the ovary most commonly originate?

    A. Breast
    B. Colon
    C. Endometrium
    D. Lung
    E. Pancreas

425. Which tumour marker(s) should be used to assess the risk of malignancy in postmenopausal ovarian cysts?

	α-Fetoprotein (AFP)	Cancer antigen 125 (CA125)	Cancer antigen 19-9 (CA19-9)	Carcinoembryonc antigen (CEA)	Lactate dehydrogenase (LDH)
A	✓	✓	✓		
B		✓			
C		✓		✓	✓
D	✓			✓	✓
E	✓		✓		✓

426. A 65-year-old woman presented with lower abdominal pain and bloating. A pelvic ultrasound scan demonstrated a complex ovarian cyst and this, with a serum CA125, gave a risk of malignancy index (RMI) score of 280.
    What further imaging is now required?

    A. CT of abdomen and pelvis
    B. CT of pelvis
    C. MRI of abdomen and pelvis
    D. MRI of pelvis
    E. Positron emission tomography (PET)-CT of thorax, abdomen and pelvis

427. For an ovarian mass to be defined as complex, one or more features need to be present.
    What are these features?

	Anechoic fluid	Papillary projections	Posterior attenuation	Complete septation/ multilocular	Solid nodules
A	✓	✓	✓		
B	✓	✓		✓	
C			✓	✓	✓
D	✓		✓		✓
E		✓		✓	✓

428. Which type of vulval intraepithelial neoplasia (VIN) is associated with the greatest risk of progression to vulval squamous cell carcinoma?

   A. Differentiated type
   B. Non-classical type
   C. Undifferentiated type
   D. Usual type (HPV-16)
   E. Warty type (HPV-2)

429. A 62-year-old woman is taking tamoxifen following surgery for breast cancer. She has experienced some vaginal bleeding. A transvaginal ultrasound scan measures her endometrial thickness as 7 mm.
   How should this be investigated?

   A. Dilation and curettage
   B. Hysteroscopy and targeted biopsy
   C. MRI scan
   D. No investigation required
   E. Pipelle endometrial biopsy

430. What is the estimated reduction in risk of ovarian cancer for each year of use of the combined oral contraceptive pill (COCP)?

   A. 2%
   B. 7%
   C. 12%
   D. 17%
   E. 22%

431. In which age group do malignant ovarian germ cell tumours (MOGCTs) most commonly occur?

   A. 0–20 years
   B. 21–40 years
   C. 41–60 years
   D. 61–80 years
   E. ≥81 years

432. A 20-year-old woman is found to have a solid ovarian mass, and tests for serum tumour markers reveal an elevated LDH. Following a multidisciplinary team discussion, there is the suspicion of a germ cell tumour.
What is the most appropriate surgical management?

	Laparo-tomy	Laparos-copy	Unilateral oophorec-tomy	Bilateral oophorec-tomy	Omental biopsy	Selective removal of lymph nodes	Systematic removal of lymph nodes
A	✓		✓		✓	✓	
B	✓			✓	✓		✓
C		✓	✓		✓	✓	
D		✓	✓				✓
E		✓		✓			✓

433. What are the two most common types of malignant ovarian germ cell tumours?

	Choriocarcinoma	Dysgerminoma	Embryonal tumour	Endodermal sinus tumour	Immature teratoma
A	✓	✓			
B	✓		✓		
C			✓	✓	
D				✓	✓
E		✓			✓

434. What is the strongest known risk factor for ovarian cancer?
A. Family history of breast cancer
B. Family history of ovarian cancer
C. Fertility treatment
D. Nulliparity
E. Smoking

435. What is the current recommendation regarding screening for ovarian cancer in women with no family history of the disease?
A. Annual calculation of RMI
B. Annual pelvic ultrasound scan
C. Annual serum CA125
D. Annual serum CA125 and pelvic ultrasound scans on alternate years
E. No screening recommended

436. For women who are carriers of a *BRCA* gene mutation and go on to have risk-reducing surgery (bilateral salpingo-oophorectomy), what is the likelihood of the subsequent development of a primary peritoneal cancer?

 A. 0.5%
 B. 2%
 C. 7%
 D. 12%
 E. 15%

437. With regard to squamous cell carcinoma of the cervix, what is believed to be the minimum time span between infection by HPV and the development of a premalignant lesion with true malignant potential?

 A. 1 year
 B. 3 years
 C. 5 years
 D. 7 years
 E. 9 years

438. What is the principle role of radiotherapy in the treatment of endometrial cancer?

 A. It is the preferred treatment option in early stage disease
 B. Postoperatively as an adjuvant therapy
 C. Postoperatively to sensitise any remaining disease to chemotherapy
 D. Preoperatively to reduce the size of large tumours
 E. There is no place for radiotherapy in the treatment of endometrial cancer

439. Which isotopes are used in modern-day brachytherapy for the treatment of gynaecological cancers?

	Caesium	Cobalt	Iridium	Radium
A	✓	✓		
B	✓		✓	
C	✓			✓
D		✓	✓	
E		✓		✓

440. Which subtype of ovarian cancer is most commonly associated with bowel obstruction?

 A. Brenner tumour
 B. Dysgerminoma
 C. Epithelial cancer
 D. Sex-cord stromal tumour
 E. Teratoma

EMQs

Options for questions 441–443

A	I A
B	I B
C	I C_1
D	I C_2
E	I C_3
F	II
G	III A_1
H	III A_2
I	III B
J	III C_1
K	III C_2
L	IV A
M	IV B

For each of the following clinical scenarios, choose the single most appropriate stage of disease from the list of options given above. Each option may be used once, more than once or not at all.

441. A 60-year-old woman has a laparoscopic bilateral oophorectomy for a persistent ovarian cyst. Her serum CA125 is 50 IU/ml. The ovarian capsule is noted to be intact, but during the course of the operation, the cyst ruptures. Peritoneal washings prior to the rupture are clear. The contralateral ovary is normal. Histology confirms an ovarian carcinoma.

442. A woman is diagnosed with cervical cancer. The carcinoma has extended into the pelvic sidewall. On rectal examination, there is no cancer-free space between the tumour and the pelvic sidewall. The tumour involves the lower third of the vagina. There is unilateral hydronephrosis.

443. A 90-year-old woman is diagnosed with vulval cancer. Imaging suggests metastases to both inguinofemoral and pelvic lymph nodes.

Options for questions 444–446

A	Cancer antigen 19-9 (CA19-9)
B	Cancer antigen 72-4 (CA72-4)
C	Carcinoembryonic antigen (CEA)
D	Epithelial tumour antigen (ETA)
E	α-Fetoprotein (AFP)
F	Homeobox protein CDX2
G	Human chorionic gonadotropin (hCG)
H	Human epididymis protein 4 (HE4)
I	Inhibin
J	Lactate dehydrogenase (LDH)
K	Oestradiol
L	Oestriol

For each of the following situations, choose the single most appropriate tumour marker from the list of options above. Each option may be chosen once, more than once or not at all.

444. A compound belonging to the transforming growth factor-β (TGF-β) superfamily, produced by both the Sertoli cells of the testis and granulosa cell tumours of the ovary.

445. A steroid that is almost undetectable in the non-pregnant female, but whose levels rise >1000-fold during pregnancy.

446. A compound that is elevated in women with an ovarian dysgerminoma.

Options for questions 447–450

A	No action necessary
B	Perform cervical cytology in 1 year's time
C	Perform cervical cytology in 3 years' time
D	Perform colposcopic treatment
E	Perform human papillomavirus (HPV) test of cure
F	Perform HPV triage testing
G	Refer to colposcopy
H	Repeat cervical cytology in 3 months' time
I	Repeat cervical cytology in 6 months' time
J	Return to routine recall

For each of the following clinical scenarios, what is the most appropriate management from the list above? Each option may be used once, more than once or not at all.

447. A 28-year-old woman attends her GP surgery for a routine cervical smear. The examination is difficult and an 'inadequate' result is returned.

448. A 35-year-old woman attends her GP surgery for a cervical smear having never had a smear in the past. A result of high-grade dyskaryosis is returned.

449. A 31-year-old woman attends her GP surgery for a cervical smear. This is reported as low-grade dyskaryosis and an HPV test is organised. Unfortunately, the HPV test is inadequate.

450. A 30-year-old woman undergoes colposcopic treatment for cervical intraepithelial neoplasia (CIN) 3. Histology shows incomplete excision at the ectocervical margin but complete excision at the endocervical margin.

Options for questions 451–453

A	15–19 years
B	20–24 years
C	25–29 years
D	30–34 years
E	35–39 years
F	40–44 years
G	45–49 years
H	50–54 years
I	55–59 years
J	60–64 years
K	65–69 years
L	70–74 years
M	75–79 years
N	80–84 years
O	85–89 years

For each of the following scenarios, choose the single most appropriate age range from the list of options above. Each option may be chosen once, more than once or not at all.

451. The age group with the highest rate of cervical cancer in the UK.

452. The age group with the highest incidence of ovarian cancer per year in the UK.

453. The age group with the highest incidence of uterine cancer per year in the UK.

Options for questions 454–456

A	1%
B	2%
C	5%
D	10%
E	20%
F	40%
G	55%
H	60%
I	70%
J	80%
K	90%
L	95%
M	100%

For each of the following cancers, choose the single most appropriate figure for the 5-year survival rate from the list of options above. Each option may be chosen once, more than once or not at all.

454. Stage 2 carcinoma of the cervix.

455. Stage 1 uterine (endometrial) cancer.

456. Stage 3 ovarian cancer.

Options for questions 457–460

A	Arrange follow-up scan in 6 months' time
B	Arrange follow-up scan in 12 months' time
C	Chemotherapy
D	Combined oral contraceptive pill (COCP) for six cycles
E	Full staging laparotomy
F	Gonadotropin-releasing hormone (GnRH) analogue for 6 months
G	Laparoscopic cyst drainage
H	Laparoscopic bilateral salpingo-oophorectomy
I	Laparoscopic ovarian cystectomy
J	Laparoscopic unilateral oophorectomy
K	Laparotomy, bilateral salpingo-oophorectomy and omental biopsy
L	Measure serum CA125 and calculate risk of malignancy index (RMI)
M	No treatment required
N	Radical hysterectomy including lymph node dissection
O	Radiotherapy
P	Sentinel node biopsy
Q	Total abdominal hysterectomy, bilateral salpingo-oophorectomy and omental biopsy
R	Ultrasound-guided cyst drainage

For each of the following clinical scenarios, choose the single most appropriate management option from the list above. Each option may be chosen once, more than once or not at all.

457. A 65-year-old woman has an incidental finding of an ovarian cyst during an MRI scan to evaluate her spine. A follow-up ultrasound confirms this to be a simple cyst with a maximum diameter of 4.5 cm. Her serum CA125 is 5 IU/l. The woman is asymptomatic.

458. A 65-year-old woman is referred urgently with weight loss, abdominal bloating and urinary urgency. An ultrasound scan demonstrates a multicystic mass with solid areas and ascites. Her serum CA125 is 100 IU/l. A CT scan confirms a suspicious mass. Which management should be recommended by the multidisciplinary team?

459. A healthy 60-year-old woman with a BMI of 28 kg/m^2 presents with lower abdominal pain and bloating. An ultrasound scan demonstrates a unilocular cyst of 4 cm diameter with a solid component. There is no ascites. Her serum CA125 is 40 IU/l.

460. A frail 90-year-old woman presents with abdominal discomfort and bloating. She has mitral stenosis and atrial fibrillation. She has urinary frequency and nocturia. An ultrasound scan reveals a 10 cm simple ovarian cyst. Her serum CA125 is 2 IU/l.

Answers

SBAs

421. Answer   **C**   Inguinal

Explanation
The natural history of vulval cancer is to grow by direct extension followed by lymphatic embolisation. Initially, this is to local inguinal lymph nodes and later to femoral and the external iliac chain.

Reference

Bailey C, Luesley D. Squamous vulval cancer – an update. *The Obstetrician & Gynaecologist* 2013;15:227–31.

422. Answer   **A**   <1%

Explanation
See Table 1 in the reference article.

Reference

Bailey C, Luesley D. Squamous vulval cancer – an update. *The Obstetrician & Gynaecologist* 2013;15:227–31.

423. Answer   **E**   Carboplatin and paclitaxel

Explanation
Surgery remains at the forefront of treatment, either as the initial therapy or as a delayed primary procedure. However, the conventional agents that continue to be used most frequently are carboplatin and paclitaxel.

Reference

Reed NS, Sadozye AH. Update on chemotherapy in gynaecological cancers. *The Obstetrician & Gynaecologist* 2016;18:182–8.

424. Answer   **C**   Endometrium

Explanation
Approximately 10% of ovarian tumours are of secondary origin. The most common metastasis is from endometrium. Krukenberg tumours commonly metastasise from the stomach or colon, although metastasis may also arise from the breast, lung and pancreas.

Reference

Sanusi FA, Carter P, Barton DPJ. Non-epithelial ovarian cancers. *The Obstetrician & Gynaecologist* 2000;2:37–9.

425. Answer   **B**   CA125

Explanation
CA125 should be the only serum tumour marker used for primary evaluation.

There is currently not enough evidence to support the routine clinical use of other tumour markers, such as human epididymis protein 4 (HE4), CEA, homeobox protein CDX2, cancer antigen 72-4 (CA72-4), CA19-9, AFP, LDH or human chorionic gonadotropin (hCG), to assess the risk of malignancy in postmenopausal ovarian cysts.

Reference

RCOG. The management of ovarian cysts in postmenopausal women. *RCOG GTG No. 34*, July 2016.

426. Answer **A** CT of abdomen and pelvis

Explanation
CT of the abdomen and pelvis should be performed for all postmenopausal women with ovarian cysts who have an RMI score of ≥200, with onward referral to a gynaecological oncology multidisciplinary team.

Reference

RCOG. The management of ovarian cysts in postmenopausal women. *RCOG GTG No. 34*, July 2016.

427. Answer **E** Papillary projections, complete septation/multilocular and/or solid nodules

Explanation
An ovarian cyst is defined as complex in the presence of one or more of the following features:

• Complete septation (i.e. multilocular cyst)
• Solid nodules
• Papillary projections.

Reference

RCOG. The management of ovarian cysts in postmenopausal women. *RCOG GTG No. 34*, July 2016.

428. Answer **A** Differentiated type

Explanation
In genitourinary medicine clinics, the commonest aetiological agent is human papillomavirus (HPV). This type of VIN is known as the usual type and is associated mainly with HPV-16. A second type, generally not HPV-related, occurs in conjunction with lichen sclerosus or lichen planus (known as differentiated type). The risk of progression to squamous cell carcinoma is much greater with the differentiated type of VIN and this needs specialised management.

Reference

Edwards SK, Bates CM, Lewis F, Sethi G, Grover D. 2014 UK national guideline on the management of vulval conditions. *International Journal of STD & AIDS* 2015;26:611–24.

429. Answer   B   Hysteroscopy and targeted biopsy

Explanation
All abnormal bleeding or spotting should be investigated, but pipelle endometrial
biopsy rarely provides useful diagnostic information in women treated with
tamoxifen; therefore, symptomatic women with a thickened endometrium should
be investigated with a hysteroscopy and targeted biopsy. This is primarily because
of tamoxifen-induced subepithelial stromal hypertrophy.

Reference

Otify M, Fuller J, Ross J, Shaikh H, Johns J. Endometrial pathology in the postmenopausal
   woman – an evidence based approach to management. *The Obstetrician & Gynaecologist*
   2015;17:29–38.

430. Answer   B   7%

Explanation
It is estimated that each year of using the COCP brings an approximate 7%
reduction in risk of ovarian cancer.

Reference

Louis LS, Saso S, Ghaem-Maghami S, Abdalla H, Smith JR. The relationship between
   infertility treatment and cancer including gynaecological cancers. *The Obstetrician &
   Gynaecologist* 2013;15:177–83.

431. Answer   A   0–20 years

Explanation
MOGCTs occur most commonly in the first two decades of life, but can appear
at any age, with 82.3% of all MOGCTs occurring between the ages of 14 and 54
years.

Reference

RCOG. Management of female malignant ovarian germ cell tumours. *RCOG Scientific
   Impact Paper No. 52*. November 2016.

**432. Answer   A   Laparotomy, unilateral oophorectomy, omental biopsy and selective
removal of lymph nodes**

Explanation
Surgery, when appropriate, should comprise unilateral oophorectomy, peritoneal
washing, omental biopsy and selective removal of enlarged lymph nodes. Biopsy
of a normal contralateral ovary is not indicated. Surgery should be by an open
procedure to enable removal of the affected ovary with its tumour intact rather
than broken or ruptured.

Reference

RCOG. Management of female malignant ovarian germ cell tumours. *RCOG Scientific
   Impact Paper No. 52*. November 2016.

433. Answer **E** Dysgerminoma and immature teratoma

Explanation
Approximately one-third of such cases are dysgerminomas, one-third are immature teratomas, and one-third include embryonal tumours, endodermal sinus tumours, choriocarcinoma and mixed-cell types.

Reference

RCOG. Management of female malignant ovarian germ cell tumours. *RCOG Scientific Impact Paper No. 52*. November 2016.

434. Answer **B** Family history of ovarian cancer

Explanation
The strongest known risk factor is a family history of the disease, which is present in about 10–15% of women with ovarian cancer.

Reference

Gaughan EMG, Walsh TA. Risk-reducing surgery for women at high risk of epithelial ovarian cancer. *The Obstetrician & Gynaecologist* 2014;16:185–91.

435. Answer **E** No screening recommended

Explanation
Screening for ovarian cancer with CA125 or ultrasound is not recommended for premenopausal and postmenopausal women without a family history of ovarian cancer. The predictive value of either test alone (<3%) yields an unacceptably high rate of false-positive results and attendant morbidity and costs.

Reference

Gaughan EMG, Walsh TA. Risk-reducing surgery for women at high risk of epithelial ovarian cancer. *The Obstetrician & Gynaecologist* 2014;16:185–91.

436. Answer **B** 2%

Explanation
It is important to remember that risk-reducing bilateral salpingo-oophorectomy is not completely protective and *BRCA* carriers still have a risk of developing primary peritoneal cancer (approximately 2% risk).

Reference

Gaughan EMG, Walsh TA. Risk-reducing surgery for women at high risk of epithelial ovarian cancer. *The Obstetrician & Gynaecologist* 2014;16:185–91.

437. Answer **D** 7 years

Explanation
Seven years is believed to be the minimum time span between infection by HPV and the development of a premalignant lesion with true malignant potential.

Reference

Aref-Adib M, Freeman-Wang T. Cervical cancer prevention and screening: the role of human papillomavirus testing. *The Obstetrician & Gynaecologist* 2016;18:251–63.

438. Answer **B** Postoperatively as an adjuvant therapy

    Explanation
    In endometrial cancer, the principal role of radiotherapy is as an adjuvant treatment postoperatively, and the past decade has seen this refined with far greater use of vagina brachytherapy and a marked reduction in the use of external beam radiotherapy.

    Reference
    Reed NS, Sadozye AH. Update on radiotherapy in gynaecological malignancies. *The Obstetrician & Gynaecologist* 2017;19:29–36.

439. Answer **D** Cobalt and iridium

    Explanation
    Over the decades, gynaecological brachytherapy has evolved from radium to caesium to modern-day cobalt and iridium sources.

    Reference
    Reed NS, Sadozye AH. Update on radiotherapy in gynaecological malignancies. *The Obstetrician & Gynaecologist* 2017;19:29–36.

440. Answer **C** Epithelial cancer

    Explanation
    While bowel obstruction is a rare presentation in women with gynaecological cancers, it is most commonly associated with ovarian cancer, the main subtype of which is epithelial ovarian cancer.

    Reference
    Kolomainen DF, Riley J, Wood J, Barton DPJ. Surgical management of bowel obstruction in gynaecological cancer. *The Obstetrician & Gynaecologist* 2017;19:63–70.

EMQs

441. Answer **C** I C_1

    This is stage I C_1 according to the International Federation of Gynecology and Obstetrics (FIGO) ovarian cancer staging classification (2014).

442. Answer **I** III B

    This is stage III B according to the FIGO staging of cervical carcinomas classification (2006).

443. Answer **M** IVB

    This is stage IV B according to the FIGO vulval cancer staging classification (2014).

444. Answer **I** Inhibin

Explanation
Inhibin supresses follicle-stimulating hormone (FSH) production and secretion by the anterior pituitary. Inhibin has been used as a tumour marker for granulosa cell tumours.

445. Answer **L** Oestriol

Explanation
The key here is to read the question properly. Although most people will answer G, hCG is not a steroid – it is a glycoprotein. Oestriol is a steroid that is produced by the placenta, and is one of the components of serum screening.

446. Answer **J** Lactate dehydrogenase (LDH)

Explanation
LDH is found throughout the body, and levels are elevated in a number of cancers. From a gynaecological perspective, it has been used as a tumour marker in ovarian dysgerminoma.

Reference

Sanusi FA, Carter P, Barton DPJ. Non-epithelial ovarian cancers. *The Obstetrician & Gynaecologist* 2000;2:37–9.

447. Answer **H** Repeat cervical cytology in 3 months' time

448. Answer **G** Refer to colposcopy

449. Answer **G** Refer to colposcopy

450. Answer **E** Perform human papillomavirus (HPV) test of cure

Explanation
See Figure 5 in the reference article.

Reference

Aref-Adib M, Freeman-Wang T. Cervical cancer prevention and screening: the role of human papillomavirus testing. *The Obstetrician & Gynaecologist* 2016;18:251–63.

451. Answer **C** 25–29 years

The incidence rates for cervical cancer in the UK for 2012–14 were highest in people aged 25–29 years.

452. Answer **M** 75–79 years

The incidence rates for ovarian cancer in the UK for 2012–14 were highest in females aged 75–79 years.

453. **Answer   L   70–74 years**

The incidence rates for uterine cancer in the UK for 2012–14 were highest in females aged 70–74 years.

Reference

See the Cancer Research UK website at www.cancerresearchuk.org (accessed 25 July 2018).

454. **Answer   G   55%**

The 5-year survival rates for stage 1 to stage 4 cervical cancer are 95.9%, 54.4%, 37.9% and 5.3%, respectively. For all stages taken together, the overall 5-year survival rate is 69.9%. Where the stage is not known, the 5-year survival rate is 31.6%.

455. **Answer   L   95%**

The 5-year survival rates for stage 1 to stage 4 uterine (endometrial) cancer are 95.3%, 77%, 39% and 13.6%,respectively. For all stages taken together, the overall 5-year survival rate is 84.4%. Where the stage is not known, the 5-year survival rate is 54.4%.

456. **Answer   E   20%**

The 5-year survival rates for stage 1 to stage 4 ovarian cancer are 90%, 42.8%, 18.6% and 3.5%, respectively. For all stages taken together, the overall 5-year survival rate is 39.3%. Where the stage is not known, the 5-year survival rate is 12.5%.

Reference

See the Cancer Research UK website at www.cancerresearchuk.org (accessed 25 July 2018).

457. **Answer   A   Arrange follow-up scan in 6 months' time**

Explanation
Asymptomatic, simple, unilateral, unilocular ovarian cysts of <5 cm in diameter have a low risk of malignancy. In the presence of normal serum CA125 levels, these cysts can be managed conservatively, with a repeat evaluation in 4–6 months. It is reasonable to discharge these women from follow-up after 1 year if the cyst remains unchanged or reduces in size, with normal serum CA125, taking into consideration the woman's wishes and surgical fitness.

458. **Answer   E   Full staging laparotomy**

Explanation
RMI is calculated as: $U \times M \times CA125$ (see question 301 for details). This woman's RMI is $3 \times 3 \times 100 = 900$.

All ovarian cysts that are suspicious of malignancy in a postmenopausal woman, as indicated by an RMI of ≥ 200, CT findings, clinical assessment or findings at laparoscopy, require a full laparotomy and staging procedure.

459. Answer   **H**   Laparoscopic bilateral salpingo-oophorectomy

Explanation
This woman's RMI is $1 \times 3 \times 40 = 120$ (see question 301 for details).

Women with an RMI of <200 (i.e. at low risk of malignancy) are suitable for laparoscopic management. Laparoscopic management of ovarian cysts in postmenopausal women should comprise bilateral salpingo-oophorectomy rather than cystectomy.

460. Answer   **R**   Ultrasound-guided cyst drainage

Explanation
This woman's RMI is $1 \times 3 \times 2 = 6$ (see question 301 for details).

This is very unlikely to be a malignant cyst, but the woman is symptomatic. She is frail with co-morbidities.

Aspiration has no role in the management of asymptomatic ovarian cysts in postmenopausal women. An exception exists for those symptomatic women who are medically unfit to undergo surgery or further intervention. In these women, aspiration will provide relief of their symptoms, albeit temporarily.

Reference

RCOG. The management of ovarian cysts in postmenopausal women. *RCOG GTG No. 34.* July 2016.

Urogynaecology and pelvic floor problems

SBAs

461. A 55-year-old woman attends the urogynaecology clinic with urinary incontinence associated with urgency. A urine dipstick is negative. A diagnosis of urgency urinary incontinence is made.

    What would be considered the first-line treatment?

    A. Bladder training
    B. Botulinum toxin A
    C. Mirabegron
    D. Oxybutynin
    E. Pelvic floor muscle training

462. A 60-year-old woman attends the urogynaecology clinic with urinary incontinence associated with coughing and sneezing. A urine dipstick is negative. A diagnosis of stress urinary incontinence is made.

    What would be considered the first-line treatment?

    A. Bladder training
    B. Desmopressin
    C. Duloxetine
    D. Systemic hormone replacement therapy (HRT)
    E. Supervised pelvic floor muscle training

463. What proportion of women who use vaginal pessaries to manage pelvic organ prolapse will report satisfaction in symptom relief?

    A. 47%
    B. 58%
    C. 69%
    D. 80%
    E. 92%

464. The incidence of asymptomatic bacteriuria in pregnancy is 2–5%.
   If untreated, what proportion of cases will proceed to lower urinary tract infection (UTI)?

   A. 20%
   B. 40%
   C. 60%
   D. 80%
   E. 90%

465. Which aetiological factor is associated with the greatest increase in risk of developing pelvic organ prolapse?

   A. Age
   B. Connective tissue disorders
   C. Menopausal status
   D. Parity
   E. Weight

466. By what factor are obese women at increased risk of anal incontinence compared with non-obese women?

   A. 2-fold
   B. 3-fold
   C. 4-fold
   D. 6-fold
   E. 8-fold

467. Which antimuscarinic drug used in the management of an overactive bladder should be avoided in frail older women?

   A. Darifenacin
   B. Desmopressin
   C. Mirabegron
   D. Oxybutynin
   E. Tolterodine

468. What is the mode of action of duloxetine?

   A. M3 receptor antagonist
   B. Monoamine oxidase inhibitor
   C. α_2-Receptor agonist
   D. β_3-Receptor agonist
   E. Serotonin–noradrenaline uptake inhibitor

469. A woman is seen on the postoperative ward round following the insertion of a transobturator tape for the treatment of stress urinary incontinence.

    Within what timeframe should she be offered a follow-up appointment with a vaginal examination to exclude erosion?

    A. Within 1 month
    B. Within 2 months
    C. Within 3 months
    D. Within 6 months
    E. Within 12 months

470. Which derangement of acid–base balance is associated with augmentation cystoplasty for the treatment of an overactive bladder?

    A. Metabolic acidosis
    B. Metabolic alkalosis
    C. No derangement
    D. Respiratory acidosis
    E. Respiratory alkalosis

471. What is the mode of action of darifenacin?

    A. M3 receptor antagonist
    B. Monoamine oxidase inhibitor
    C. α_2-Receptor agonist
    D. β_3-Receptor agonist
    E. Serotonin–noradrenaline uptake inhibitor

472. Following a vaginal hysterectomy, it is noted that the vaginal vault is at the level of the introitus.

    What further surgical procedure would be advised?

    A. Anterior repair
    B. McCall culdoplasty
    C. Moschcowitz procedure
    D. Sacrocolpopexy
    E. Sacrospinous fixation

473. Which invasive treatment for an overactive bladder is suitable for women who are unable to perform clean intermittent catheterisation?

    A. Augmentation cystoplasty
    B. Botulinum toxin A
    C. Detrusor myomectomy
    D. Percutaneous sacral nerve stimulation
    E. Transobturator tape

474. In the pelvic organs prolapse quantification (POP-Q) examination, what is the description of Aa?
   A. Anterior vaginal wall at the level of the hymen
   B. Anterior vaginal wall 1 cm proximal to the hymen
   C. Anterior vaginal wall 2 cm proximal to the hymen
   D. Anterior vaginal wall 3 cm proximal to the hymen
   E. Anterior wall 4 cm proximal to the hymen

475. Colpocleisis is a safe and effective procedure that can be considered for frail women and/or women who do not wish to retain sexual function.
   What proportion of cases of colpocleisis that are performed would be considered successful?
   A. 17%
   B. 37%
   C. 57%
   D. 77%
   E. 97%

476. What factor is most likely to aggravate the pain in patients with bladder pain syndrome?
   A. Coffee
   B. Constrictive clothing
   C. Sexual intercourse
   D. Spicy foods
   E. Stress

477. What proportion of patients with bladder pain syndrome will get relief of symptoms from voiding?
   A. 17–28%
   B. 31–42%
   C. 44–56%
   D. 57–73%
   E. 78–92%

478. What is the most common problem for a woman following cystoscopy?
   A. Bladder perforation requiring catheterisation
   B. Mild burning or bleeding during micturition
   C. Significant haematuria requiring clot evacuation
   D. UTI
   E. Urinary retention requiring catheterisation

479. What is the only true contraindication to cystoscopy?

    A. Congenital urinary tract anomalies
    B. Untreated UTI
    C. Urethral stricture
    D. Vesicovaginal fistula
    E. Visible haematuria

480. What is the risk of developing a pelvic abscess following a vaginal hysterectomy for uterovaginal prolapse?

    A. 1 in 1000 women
    B. 2 in 1000 women
    C. 3 in 1000 women
    D. 4 in 1000 women
    E. 5 in 1000 women

EMQs

Options for questions 481–483

A	Abdominal X-ray
B	Bladder scan
C	Complete a bladder diary
D	CT of pelvis
E	Cystoscopy
F	Digital assessment of pelvic floor contraction
G	Filling and voiding cystometry
H	MRI of pelvis
I	No investigation required
J	Pad testing
K	Pelvic ultrasound scan
L	Perform a quality-of-life assessment
M	Repeat midstream urine
N	Ultrasound scan of renal tract
O	Urinary catheterisation
P	Urine dipstick test
Q	Video urodynamics

For each of the following clinical scenarios, what is the most appropriate investigation that needs to be performed before any therapy is commenced? Each option may be used once, more than once or not at all.

481. A 40-year-old woman attends the gynaecology clinic with a history of leakage of urine on coughing or sneezing following the birth of her last child 2 years ago. A urine dipstick is negative. A decision is made to commence a course of supervised pelvic floor muscle training.

482. A 55-year-old woman who previously had insertion of a tension-free vaginal tape for the treatment of stress incontinence attends with new symptoms of urinary leakage with physical exertion or coughing. She is requesting further surgery.

483. A 60-year-old woman has an initial appointment at the gynaecology clinic. Her presenting symptoms are urinary leakage, urgency and nocturia.

Options for questions 484–486

A	Botulinum toxin A
B	Botulinum toxin B
C	Darifenacin
D	Desmopressin
E	Dimethyl sulfoxide
F	Duloxetine
G	Flavoxate
H	Imipramine
I	Mirabegron
J	Oestriol cream
K	Oxybutynin
L	Propantheline
M	Propiverine
N	Solifenacin
O	Tibolone
P	Tolterodine
Q	Transdermal oestrogen
R	Trospium

For each of the following clinical scenarios, choose the single most appropriate pharmacological therapy from the list above. Each option may be used once, more than once or not at all.

484. A 60-year-old woman returns to the urogynaecology clinic for a review. She initially presented with symptoms of urinary leakage and urgency. She has completed a course of bladder training with no effect. She has myasthenia gravis but is otherwise well.

485. A 55-year-old woman initially presented with urinary leakage on coughing and sneezing. She completed a course of pelvic floor muscle training with little effect. She wishes to avoid surgical intervention.

486. A 62-year-old woman who is otherwise fit and well presents with urgency, urinary leakage and nocturia. The urgency and leakage are improved with transdermal oxybutynin, but the nocturia remains troublesome with her needing to go to the toilet four or five times per night.

Options for questions 487–489

A	Berger's disease (IgA nephropathy)
B	Bladder calculus
C	Bladder endometriosis
D	Cystocele
E	Foreign body
F	Haemophilia A
G	Idiopathic haematuria
H	Paroxysmal nocturnal haemoglobinuria
I	Polycystic kidney disease
J	Poststreptococcal glomerulonephritis
K	Renal calculus
L	Sickle-cell disease
M	Transitional cell carcinoma
N	Urethrocele
O	Urinary tract infection (UTI)
P	Von Willebrand's disease

For each of the following clinical scenarios, choose the single most likely cause of haematuria. Each option may be used once, more than once or not at all.

487. A 25-year-old woman presents to her GP with urinary frequency and dysuria. Her urine dipstick results are:

Leucocytes	+
Nitrites	+
Blood	+++
Protein	+
Ketones	−
Glucose	−

488. Two days after an upper respiratory tract infection, a 20-year-old woman presents to her GP with episodes of frank haematuria. Renal function tests are normal.

489. A 45-year-old woman presents with acute loin pain and haematuria. She is found to be hypertensive with abnormal renal function tests.

Options for questions 490–492

A	Anterior and posterior colporrhaphy
B	Anterior colporrhaphy
C	Artificial urinary sphincter
D	Augmentation cystoplasty
E	Colpocleisis
F	Fenton's procedure
G	Intramural bulking agents
H	Laparoscopic colposuspension
I	Marshall–Marchetti–Krantz procedure
J	Open colposuspension
K	Posterior colporrhaphy
L	Tension-free vaginal tape
M	Transobturator tape
N	Urinary diversion
O	Vaginal hysterectomy

For each of the following clinical scenarios, choose the single most appropriate surgical intervention from the list of options above. Each option may be used once, more than once or not at all.

490. A woman attends the urogynaecology clinic with symptoms of stress incontinence that have not responded to conservative measures. She is keen for surgical intervention but wishes to avoid synthetic meshes and tapes as she has read adverse reports in the media.

491. A 45-year-old woman presents with urinary frequency and urgency and a diagnosis of idiopathic detrusor overactivity is made. This has not responded to conservative measures and she is ready to proceed with surgical intervention.

492. A 90-year-old woman with hypertension and type 2 diabetes presents with worsening uterovaginal prolapse that is not being controlled with shelf pessaries.

Options for questions 493 and 494

A	Atrophic vaginitis
B	Bladder calculus
C	Bladder diverticulum
D	Bladder endometriosis
E	Bladder pain syndrome
F	Fibromyalgia
G	Pelvic inflammatory disease (PID)
H	Peritoneal adhesions
I	Sjögren's syndrome
J	Systemic lupus erythematosus
K	Transitional cell carcinoma
L	Urethral diverticulum
M	Urinary tract infection (UTI)
N	Vesicovaginal fistula

For each of the following clinical scenarios, choose the single most likely diagnosis from the list of options above. Each option may be used once, more than once or not at all.

493. A 40-year-old woman with no significant past medical history presents with a 10-month history of pelvic pain mainly located to the suprapubic area. She has urinary urgency and frequency but no leakage. The symptoms persist through her cycle. She suffers with constipation but not diarrhoea.

494. A 48-year-old woman presents to clinic with complex symptoms. She has urinary urgency and frequency but also dysuria and postmicturition dribble. A full gynaecological history also reveals dyspareunia. An initial pelvic examination is unremarkable.

Options for questions 495–497

A	Arrange CT of kidneys, ureters and bladder (CT KUB)
B	Arrange MRI scan
C	Complete bladder diary
D	Consider antibiotics while awaiting midstream urine culture results
E	Measure postvoid residual volume by bladder scan
F	Measure postvoid residual volume by catheterisation
G	Perform cystoscopy
H	Perform digital pelvic examination
I	Perform pad test
J	Perform urodynamic testing
K	Prescribe antibiotics while awaiting midstream urine culture results
L	Refer to urologist
M	Send urine for culture and sensitivity

From the list of management options above, choose the single most appropriate management for each of the following clinical scenarios. Each option may be used once, more than once or not at all.

495. A woman attends a general gynaecology clinic and has routine urinalysis by dipstick. She has no symptoms, but the urine tests positive for both leucocytes and nitrites.

496. A woman is referred to a urogynaecologist with recurrent UTIs. A urine dipstick in the clinic is negative.

497. A 53-year-old woman is referred to the urogynaecology clinic with urinary incontinence. She has routine urine dipstick testing and is found to have microscopic haematuria.

Options for questions 498–500

A	Bulbospongiosus muscle
B	Conjoint longitudinal coat
C	External anal sphincter
D	Iliococcygeus
E	Internal anal sphincter
F	Ischial tuberosities
G	Ischiocavernosus muscle
H	Ischiococcygeus muscle
I	Ischiopubic rami
J	Levator ani
K	Levator hiatus
L	Puborectalis muscle
M	Pubovaginalis muscle
N	Sacrotuberous ligaments
O	Superficial transverse perineal muscles

From the list of options above, choose the single most appropriate anatomical structure from the list of descriptions below. Each option may be used once, more than once or not at all.

498. The most caudal component of the levator ani complex.

499. The structure separating the external and internal anal sphincters.

500. The structure accounting for the majority of the resting anal pressure.

Answers

SBAs

461. **Answer A Bladder training**

Explanation
Offer bladder training lasting for a minimum of 6 weeks as the first-line treatment to women with urgency or mixed urinary incontinence.

Reference
NICE. Urinary incontinence in women: management. *NICE Clinical Guideline (CG 171)*. September 2013.

462. **Answer E Supervised pelvic floor muscle training**

Explanation
Offer a trial of supervised pelvic floor muscle training of at least 3 months' duration as the first-line treatment to women with stress or mixed urinary incontinence.

Reference
NICE. Urinary incontinence in women: management. *NICE Clinical Guideline (CG 171)*. September 2013.

463. **Answer E 92%**

Explanation
Women have used mechanical devices to reduce pelvic organ prolapse since ancient times, and the use of vaginal pessaries remains a simple and satisfactory treatment. One study of 100 women using this method showed a 92% satisfaction rate in terms of prolapse symptoms.

Reference
Jefferis H, Jackson SR, Price N. Management of uterine prolapse: is hysterectomy necessary? *The Obstetrician & Gynaecologist* 2016;18:17–23.

464. **Answer A 20%**

Explanation
The incidence of asymptomatic bacteriuria during pregnancy is 2–5%, and if not treated, up to 20% of women will develop a lower UTI.

Reference
Asali F, Mahfouz I, Phillips C. The management of urogynaecological problems in pregnancy and the early postpartum period. *The Obstetrician & Gynaecologist* 2012;14:153–8.

465. **Answer D Parity**

Explanation
Parity is associated with the greatest increase in risk of developing pelvic organ prolapse.

Reference

Asali F, Mahfouz I, Phillips C. The management of urogynaecological problems in pregnancy and the early postpartum period. *The Obstetrician & Gynaecologist* 2012;14:153–8.

466. **Answer   A   2-fold**

Explanation

Obesity appears to confer a 4-fold and 2-fold increased risk of urinary and anal incontinence, respectively.

Reference

Jain P, Parsons M. The effects of obesity on the pelvic floor. *The Obstetrician & Gynaecologist* 2011;13:133–42.

467. **Answer   D   Oxybutynin**

Explanation

Do not offer oxybutynin (immediate release) to frail older women.

Reference

NICE. Urinary incontinence in women: management. *NICE Clinical Guideline (CG171)*. September 2013.

468. **Answer   E   Serotonin–noradrenaline uptake inhibitor**

Explanation

Duloxetine is a combined serotonin and noradrenaline reuptake inhibitor. Adverse effects are largely related to increases in levels of noradrenaline and serotonin, and include gastrointestinal disturbances, dry mouth, headache, decreased libido and anorgasmia.

Reference

Orme S, Ramsay I. Duloxetine: the long awaited drug treatment for stress urinary incontinence. *The Obstetrician & Gynaecologist* 2005;7:117–19.

469. **Answer   D   Within 6 months**

Explanation

Offer a follow-up appointment (including a vaginal examination to exclude erosion) within 6 months to all women who have had continence surgery.

Reference

NICE. Urinary incontinence in women: management. *NICE Clinical Guideline (CG171)*. September 2013.

470. **Answer   A   Metabolic acidosis**

Explanation

Before augmentation cystoplasty, preoperative counselling for the woman or her carer should include the common and serious complications: bowel disturbance, metabolic acidosis, mucus production and/or retention in the bladder, UTI and urinary retention.

Reference

NICE. Urinary incontinence in women: management. *NICE Clinical Guideline (CG171).* September 2013.

471. Answer   **A**   M3 receptor antagonist

Explanation
See Table 1 in the reference article.

Reference

Abboudi H, Fynes MM, Doumouchtsis SK. Contemporary therapy for the overactive bladder. *The Obstetrician & Gynaecologist* 2011;13:98–106.

472. Answer   **E**   Sacrospinous fixation

Explanation
Sacrospinous fixation is recommended if the vaginal vault is at the introitus at the end of a vaginal hysterectomy procedure.

Reference

RCOG/BSUG. Post-hysterectomy vaginal vault prolapse. *RCOG GTG No. 46.* July 2015.

473. Answer   **D**   Percutaneous sacral nerve stimulation

Explanation
Offer percutaneous sacral nerve stimulation to women after a multidisciplinary team review if:

- Their overactive bladder has not responded to conservative management including drugs and
- They are unable to perform clean intermittent catheterisation.

Start treatment with botulinum toxin A only if the woman has been trained in clean intermittent catheterisation and has performed the technique successfully.

Restrict augmentation cystoplasty for the management of idiopathic detrusor overactivity to women whose condition has not responded to conservative management and who are willing and able to self-catheterise.

Reference

NICE. Urinary incontinence in women: management. *NICE Clinical Guideline (CG171).* September 2013.

474. Answer   **D**   Anterior vaginal wall 3 cm proximal to the hymen

Explanation
See Appendix 1 in the reference article.

Reference

RCOG/BSUG. Post-hysterectomy vaginal vault prolapse. *RCOG GTG No. 46.* July 2015.

475. Answer **E** 97%

Explanation
Colpocleisis has a short operating time and a low incidence of complications. One published study included 33 women and a second included 92 women. Success rates of ≥97% have been reported.

Reference
RCOG/BSUG. Post-hysterectomy vaginal vault prolapse. *RCOG GTG No. 46*. July 2015.

476. Answer **E** Stress

Explanation
A study of 565 patients with bladder pain syndrome was used to identify factors that can aggravate and alleviate this condition. Pain was found to be aggravated by stress (61%), sexual intercourse (50%), constrictive clothing (49%), acidic beverages (54%), coffee (51%) and spicy foods (46%).

Reference
RCOG. Management of bladder pain syndrome. *RCOG GTG No. 70*. December 2016.

477. Answer **D** 57–73%

Explanation
In a study of 565 patients with bladder pain syndrome, voiding was found to relieve the pain in 57–73% of patients.

Reference
RCOG. Management of bladder pain syndrome. *RCOG GTG No. 70*. December 2016.

478. Answer **B** Mild burning or bleeding during micturition

Explanation
The risks associated with cystoscopy in women are as follows:
Common risks (>1 in 10):
- Mild burning or bleeding on passing urine for a short period after the operation
- Biopsy of abnormal areas in bladder.

Occasional risks (between 1 in 10 and 1 in 50):
- Infection of the bladder requiring antibiotics.

Rare risks (<1 in 50):
- Temporary insertion of a catheter
- Delayed bleeding requiring removal of clots or further surgery
- Injury to the urethra causing delayed scar formation
- Very rarely, perforation of the bladder requiring a temporary catheter or open surgical repair.

Reference

Lyttle M, Fowler G. Cystoscopy for the gynaecologist: how to do a cystoscopy. *The Obstetrician & Gynaecologist* 2017;19:236–40.

479. Answer   **B**   Untreated UTI

Explanation
The only true contraindication to cystoscopy is an untreated UTI, as outlined in the British Association of Urological Surgeons (BAUS) guidelines.

Reference

Lyttle M, Fowler G. Cystoscopy for the gynaecologist: how to do a cystoscopy. *The Obstetrician & Gynaecologist* 2017;19:236–40.

480. Answer   **C**   3 in 1000 women

Explanation
The risk of a pelvic abscess is 3 in every 1000 women (uncommon).

Reference

RCOG. Vaginal surgery for prolapse. *RCOG Consent Advice No. 5.* October 2009.

EMQs

481. Answer   **F**   Digital assessment of pelvic floor contraction

Explanation
Undertake routine digital assessment to confirm pelvic floor muscle contraction before the use of supervised pelvic floor muscle training for the treatment of urinary incontinence.

482. Answer   **G**   Filling and voiding cystometry

Explanation
After undertaking a detailed clinical history and examination, perform multichannel filling and voiding cystometry before surgery in women who have had previous surgery for stress incontinence.

483. Answer   **P**   Urine dipstick test

Explanation
Undertake a urine dipstick test in all women presenting with urinary incontinence to detect the presence of blood, glucose, protein, leucocytes and nitrites in the urine.

Reference

NICE. Urinary incontinence in women: management. *NICE Clinical Guideline (CG171).* September 2013.

484. Answer **I** Mirabegron

Explanation
Mirabegron is recommended as an option for treating the symptoms of an overactive bladder only for people in whom antimuscarinic drugs are contraindicated or clinically ineffective, or have unacceptable side effects.
Myasthenia gravis is a contraindication to antimuscarinics.

Reference
NICE. Mirabegron for treating symptoms of overactive bladder. *NICE Technology Appraisal Guidance (TA290).* June 2013.

485. Answer **F** Duloxetine

Explanation
Do not routinely offer duloxetine as a second-line treatment for women with stress urinary incontinence, although it may be offered as second-line therapy if women prefer pharmacological to surgical treatment or are not suitable for surgical treatment. If duloxetine is prescribed, counsel women about its adverse effects.

486. Answer **D** Desmopressin

Explanation
The use of desmopressin may be considered specifically to reduce nocturia in women with urinary incontinence or an overactive bladder who find it a troublesome symptom. Use particular caution in women with cystic fibrosis and avoid in those >65 years with cardiovascular disease or hypertension.

Reference
NICE. Urinary incontinence in women: management. *NICE Clinical Guideline (CG171).* September 2013.

487. Answer **O** Urinary tract infection (UTI)

Explanation
Urinary frequency or dysuria suggests a UTI, which is the most common cause of haematuria in young women.

488. Answer **A** Berger's disease (IgA nephropathy)

Explanation
IgA nephropathy is the most common glomerulonephritis worldwide and tends to present in young adults within a few days of an upper respiratory tract infection. Poststreptococcal glomerulonephritis would tend to present much later.

489. Answer   **I**   Polycystic kidney disease

Explanation
Autosomal-dominant polycystic kidney disease is the most common inherited kidney disorder. Renal dysfunction may not present until after 40 years of age but is often associated with hypertension. A renal calculus may give similar symptoms but would not be associated with hypertension and abnormal renal function tests.

Reference

Price N, Jackson S. *Urogynaecology for the MRCOG and Beyond.* 2nd edn. Cambridge: Cambridge University Press, 2012.

490. Answer   **J**   Open colposuspension

Explanation
If conservative management for stress urinary incontinence has failed, offer one of the following:

- A synthetic midurethral tape
- Open colposuspension
- An autologous rectus fascial sling.

Reference

NICE. Urinary incontinence in women: management. *NICE Clinical Guideline (CG171).* September 2013.

491. Answer   **D**   Augmentation cystoplasty

Explanation
Restrict augmentation cystoplasty for the management of idiopathic detrusor overactivity to women whose condition has not responded to conservative management and who are willing and able to self-catheterise.

Reference

NICE. Urinary incontinence in women: management. *NICE Clinical Guideline (CG171).* September 2013.

492. Answer   **E**   Colpocleisis

Explanation
Colpocleisis is often reserved for elderly patients, in particular those with co-morbidities that may render them unsuitable for the longer operating times and more invasive procedures associated with reconstructive surgery.

Reference

Jefferis H, Jackson SR, Price N. Management of uterine prolapse: is hysterectomy necessary? *The Obstetrician & Gynaecologist* 2016;18:17–23.

493. Answer **E** Bladder pain syndrome

Explanation
The widespread definition for bladder pain syndrome is that proposed by the European Society for the Study of BPS (ESSIC) in 2008 as 'pelvic pain, pressure or discomfort perceived to be related to the bladder, lasting at least 6 months, and accompanied by at least one other urinary symptom, for example persistent urge to void or frequency, in the absence of other identifiable causes'.

Reference
RCOG. Management of bladder pain syndrome. *RCOG GTG No. 70.* December 2016.

494. Answer **L** Urethral diverticulum

Explanation
A urethral diverticulum may present with multiple symptoms. The historical classical triad of dysuria, postvoid dribbling and dyspareunia is only seen in a minority of patients. Lower urinary tract symptoms, namely frequency and urgency, are present in 40–100% of cases.

Reference
Archer R, Blackman J, Stott M, Barrington J. Urethral diverticulum. *The Obstetrician & Gynaecologist* 2015;17:125–9.

495. Answer **M** Send urine for culture and sensitivity

Explanation
If women do not have symptoms of a UTI but their urine tests positive for both leucocytes and nitrites, do not offer antibiotics without the results of a midstream urine culture.

496. Answer **E** Measure postvoid residual volume by bladder scan

Explanation
Measure the postvoid residual volume by a bladder scan or catheterisation in women with symptoms suggestive of voiding dysfunction or recurrent UTIs. A bladder scan is used in preference to catheterisation on the grounds of acceptability and a lower incidence of adverse events.

497. Answer **L** Refer to urologist

Explanation
Urgently refer women with urinary incontinence who have any of the following:
- Microscopic haematuria in women aged ≥50 years
- Visible haematuria
- Recurrent or persisting UTI associated with haematuria in women aged ≥40 years
- A suspected malignant mass arising from the urinary tract.

Reference

NICE. Urinary incontinence in women: management. *NICE Clinical Guideline (CG171)*. September 2013.

498. Answer   **L**   Puborectalis muscle

Explanation
The puborectalis muscle is the most caudal component of the levator ani complex and is situated cephalad to the deep component of the external anal sphincter, from which it is almost inseparable.

499. Answer   **B**   Conjoint longitudinal coat

Explanation
The anal sphincter complex consists of the external and internal anal sphincters separated by the conjoint longitudinal coat.

500. Answer   **E**   Internal anal sphincter

Explanation
The internal anal sphincter is innervated by the sympathetic (L5) and parasympathetic (S2–S4) nerves and accounts for 50–85% of the resting anal pressure.

Reference

Lone F, Sultan A, Thakar R. Obstetric pelvic floor and anal sphincter injuries. *The Obstetrician & Gynaecologist* 2012;14:257–66.

Index